HERBAL REMEDIES FOR BEGINNERS

Unlock the Healing Powers of Holistic Antibiotics, Natural Medicine, and Forgotten Herbalism for Peace of Body and Mind

JANE KENNEDY

TABLE OF CONTENTS

Introduction 1

Chapter 1 4

Introduction to Herbal Medicine 4

History of Herbal Medicine 5

    Ancient Practices 5

    Evolution Through History 5

    Integration With Modern Medicine 6

    Herbal Medicine Today 7

Key Concepts in Herbal Healing 7

    The Concept of the Energetics of Herbs 8

    Synergy of Ingredients 8

    Individualization 9

Benefits of Herbal Remedies 10

    Affordability 10

    Fewer Side Effects 11

    Promoting Preventive Care 11

    Cultural and Personal Connection to Nature and Individual Health 12

Chapter 2 13

Starting Your Herbal Journey 13

Essential Tools for Herbal Preparation 14

    The Necessities 14

    Next Level 15

Cleaning and Maintenance 16

Your Workspace...16

Reliable Sources for Herbal Education 17

Books and Literature 17

Online Courses and Workshops 17

Herbalist Communities and Organizations 18

Podcasts and Blogs..18

Creating Your First Herbal Toolkit..18

Choosing Essential Herbs 19

Storage Solutions 19

Herbal Recipes for Beginners 20

Regular Reassessment of the Toolkit....................................21

Chapter 3 ....**23**

Popular Herbs and Their Uses **23**

Top Herbs for Beginners..23

Lavender...24

Peppermint 24

Chamomile 24

Echinacea 25

Basil 25

Lemon Balm...26

Rosemary 26

Turmeric..26

Ginger..27

Thyme 27

Ginseng 27

Properties and Benefits of the Herbs 28

Antioxidant 28

Anti-inflammatory 28

Immune Boosting 28

Cognitive Function 29

Incorporation 29

Common Conditions 30

Nausea and Digestive Issues 30

Respiratory Health 32

Anxiety and Stress 33

Skincare 33

Growing and Harvesting Tips 34

Harvesting Methods 34

Storing 34

Pest Management 35

Growing Indoors 35

Watering and Soil Fertility 35

Experimentation 36

When to Stop 36

Chapter 4 .... **38**

Herbal Preparation Methods **38**

Making Herbal Teas and Infusions 38

Steeping Time and Temperature 39

Flavor Enhancing 39

Safety Considerations 40

Preparing Tinctures and Extracts 40

Alcohol-Based Tincture 41

Preparation Steps: 41

Non-Alcoholic Tincture 41

Storing Tinctures 43

Crafting Salves and Balms 43

Oil Infusion 45

Drying and Storing Herbs Properly 46

Drying Herbs...46

Storing 47

Labeling 47

Keeping Track...47

Chapter 5 ....**49**

Daily Health Maintenance...**49**

Herbs for Boosting Immunity 49

Elderberry..50

Garlic...50

Andrographis...50

Incorporation 51

Herbs for Stress Relief and Relaxation 52

Calming Lavender..52

Anxiety-Reducing Lemon Balm 53

Sedative Passionflower 53

Enhancing Sleep With Herbal Remedies 54

Valerian Root 54

Hops 54

Magnolia Bark...55

The Return of Chamomile 55

Herbal Antibiotics 56

Echinacea 57

Goldenseal 57

Thyme and Oregano 57

How It Works 58

Chapter 6 .... **60**

Targeted Treatments **60**

Managing Pain and Inflammation 60

Turmeric 61

Willow Bark 61

Ginger 62

Devil's Claw 62

Incorporation 63

Herbal Support for Respiratory Health 63

Thyme 64

Peppermint 64

Eucalyptus 64

Lobelia 65

Natural Remedies for Skin Conditions 66

Aloe Vera 66

Calendula 67

Tea Tree Oil 67

Lavender in Short 68

Using Herbs for Women's Health 68

Chaste Tree Berry (Vitex) 68

Red Clover 69

Evening Primrose Oil 69

Nettle 70

Integrating Herbal Remedies Into Daily Routines 70

Chapter 7 ....**72**

Safety and Contraindications **72**

Potential Side Effects and Allergies...............................73

Understanding Allergic Reactions to Herbal Remedies...........73

Typical Side Effects of Herbal Remedies 73

Assessing Risk Factors...74

What to Do if You Experience a Reaction......................74

Building Awareness and Seeking Professional Guidance 75

Interactions With Pharmaceutical Medications 75

Timing 76

Safe Dosages and Administration Guidelines.............................77

Understanding Dosage Principles 77

Common Dosage Forms..77

Signs of Overdose 78

Consulting Professional Resources 78

Practical Guidelines for Safe Dosage.............................79

Importance of Professional Guidance 80

Support System 81

Chapter 8 ....**83**

Sustainable Herbal Practices **83**

Sustainable Harvesting Techniques 83

Foraging Laws...83

Best Practices for Harvesting 84

Good Agricultural Practices (GAP) 86

Supporting Ethical Herb Suppliers................................... 86

Ethical Suppliers 87

Fair Trade and Organic Farming................................... 87

Local Businesses and Directly Engaging With Suppliers 87

Advocating for Change 88

Growing Your Own Herbs Organically 89

Organic 89

Pest Control 89

Water Conservation... 89

Limited Space... 90

Attention and Care 90

Contributing to Biodiversity Preservation...................... 91

Understanding Biodiversity... 91

Native vs. Non-Native Species....................................... 92

Planting for Pollinators... 92

Community Involvement in Preservation 93

Chapter 9.. **95**

Integrating Herbs Into Modern Life.................................. **95**

Blending Herbal Traditions With Modern Medicine 95

Utilizing Herbs in Everyday Cooking 97

Creating an Herbal Home Apothecary 98

Essential Herbs for a Home Apothecary 98

Storage and Organization Tips....................................... 99

Understanding Basic Herbal Preparation Techniques........... 100

Routine Maintenance of Your Apothecary 101

Developing Personal Herbal Rituals 101

The Future of Herbal Integration 102

Conclusion..**105**

Glossary...**107**

References **110**

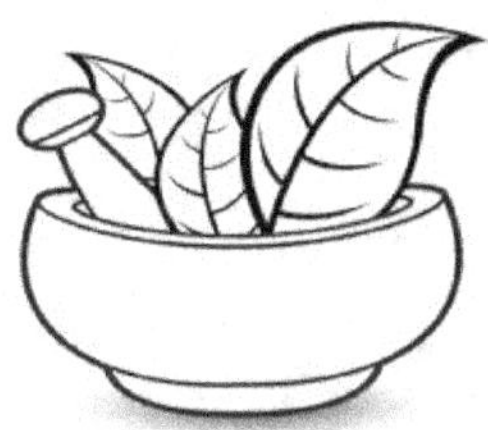

INTRODUCTION

Have you ever contemplated how our ancestors treated injuries and healed wounds with the help of humble plants, or pondered what secrets nature holds for modern ailments? Pondered the mysteries that the natural world offers us? Embarking on an exploration of herbal medicine starts with nothing but a spark of curiosity and an eagerness to uncover nature's treasures.

Today, as we navigate through an era dominated by advanced pharmaceutical solutions, we are seeing a noticeable shift in health approaches as more people turn back to natural methods for their well-being. This change reflects a growing understanding of the side effects that can come with synthetic medications. Many individuals are now exploring natural alternatives, finding comfort in herbal remedies that have supported health and wellness for generations. Whether it is easing stress or alleviating minor discomforts, these traditional solutions and remedies are being respected and valued once again.

Even though herbal treatments have a rich history and clear advantages, they frequently face doubt. A lot of people think that learning about and utilizing herbs is something only experts can do and that this expertise and knowledge is reserved for professionals. Yet, this could not be more wrong. With the proper support and guidance, anyone can embrace herbal medicine, for it is accessible to most of us. It offers a gentle and powerful way to improve our health and by clearing up these misunderstandings, we can take a holistic path to wellness that is both liberating and fulfilling.

As we move forward into the coming chapters of this book, we will dive into an exciting adventure together where we will uncover the history of herbal medicine, learn how to craft and prepare your own remedies, and find ways to incorporate these remarkable herbs into your everyday routines. This book will be your companion, blending time-honored traditions with cutting-edge findings and providing you with real-world advice and practical strategies. By the end of this journey, you will walk away with not just knowledge, but a heartfelt bond to the natural world that envelops us.

Merely picture feeling confident in your ability to make informed choices about your health, how could it make your life different in a positive sense? Perhaps it would look something like waking up each morning knowing that you can make decisions that will positively impact your well-being. This feeling of assurance can change so many aspects of your life if you allow for it to do so. For then, you will be able to approach everyday situations with a positive mindset where you can enjoy your daily activities without the nagging doubt about whether you are doing the right thing for your body.

Empowerment lies in education, and by educating yourself about herbal remedies, you are taking proactive steps towards better health. This journey is about more than just remedies; it's about reclaiming your health and becoming attuned to your body's needs. As nature offers a bounty of healing, waiting to be embraced, where each herb tells a story of tradition, healing, and the interconnectedness of all living things—you are merely steps away from changing your life. Together, we will uncover these age-old truths throughout the pages of this book and your newfound knowledge will transform the way you view your environment, nurturing a deep love for the delicate balance and beauty found in the natural world.

Whether you have a green thumb or have never planted a seed, the world of herbal remedies is open to you and will be for as long as you invite into your life. Simple preparation methods and readily available herbs make the journey beginner friendly. With step-by-step instructions and detailed explanations, you will find that incorporating herbal remedies into your routine is much simpler than you might have imagined. This book will arm you with the tools needed to start experimenting with confidence, thus ensuring that even the novice herbalist can feel competent and assured in their practice.

The intention is that each chapter will pique your curiosity and invite you to experiment with different herbs, flavors, and applications—awakening your inner herbalist. The process of exploring and creating your own remedies is not only educational but also incredibly gratifying, as you will soon get to experience it firsthand. You will discover the joy of crafting personalized solutions that are tailored to your individual needs, and in doing so, enhancing your connection to the healing properties of plants.

Take the first step of this exciting journey now; turn the pages and allow your curiosity to guide you. While you embrace the wisdom of age-old customs, the usefulness of contemporary techniques, and the deep bond we share with the natural world, your exploration will not only enrich your knowledge but also transform your approach to health and reshape how you view wellness.

By understanding and utilizing the art of herbal medicine, you are not only nurturing yourself but also contributing to a broader movement. A movement that is working towards holistic health, sustainability, and a deeper respect for the natural world. So, welcome to the world of herbal remedies—a wonderous and magical dimension of life, where every leaf, root, and flower holds the potential to heal and inspire.

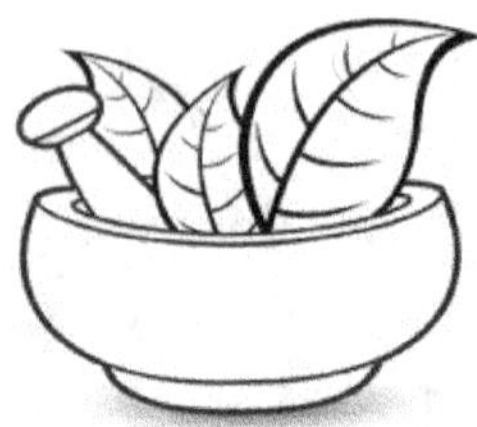

CHAPTER 1

Introduction to Herbal Medicine

Understanding and getting deep insight into the world of herbal medicine involves exploring a practice that has been rooted in human history for thousands of years. This chapter aims to introduce you to the foundational principles of this ancient yet continually evolving field, this ancient craft that grows and shifts alongside our understanding of health. From the early days when Egyptian healers skillfully harnessed the powers of humble plants like garlic and juniper, to the advanced incorporation of herbs in Traditional Chinese Medicine and Ayurveda, the use of plants in healing has been a common thread across many cultures. Herbal medicine isn't merely a thing of the past; it is a vibrant, living practice that evolves with each new scientific revelation, for it blends age-old wisdom with contemporary methods to craft a holistic pathway to wellness. For many, this offers a refreshing alternative to conventional treatments and therefore resonates deeply with those in pursuit of natural healing options.

Throughout this chapter we will explore the history and evolution of herbal medicine, emphasizing ancient healing practices and their relevance today. You will be introduced to key concepts like holistic approaches and herbal synergy, understand the benefits of herbal remedies, and gain the knowledge to incorporate these natural treatments into your own life for better health.

History of Herbal Medicine

Ancient Practices

Herbal medicine, one of the oldest forms of treatment known to humanity, has been used for thousands of years across various cultures. In ancient Egypt, healers harnessed the power of plants like garlic and juniper, documented extensively in the Ebers Papyrus—a medical text dating back to 1550 BCE (Wachtel-Galor & Benzie, 2011). The Greeks contributed significantly with figures such as Hippocrates, often referred to as the father of medicine. He advocated for the use of herbal treatments based on a deep understanding of the body's natural healing processes. Meanwhile, Traditional Chinese Medicine (TCM) has incorporated herbs into its practices for over 2,500 years, utilizing remedies such as ginseng and ephedra to balance the body's energy flow or "qi" (Wachtel-Galor & Benzie, 2011).

Similarly, India's traditional system of medicine, Ayurveda, integrates herbs like turmeric and ashwagandha for their health-promoting properties. Native American tribes also relied heavily on local flora, using plants like echinacea and sage to treat various ailments. This vast historical web reveals how integral plants have always been integrated in the quest for health (World Health Organization, 2023).

Evolution Through History

As civilizations advanced, so did their use and understanding of herbal medicine. During the Middle Ages, monasteries became centers of medicinal knowledge, preserving and synthesizing information from ancient texts. European herbalists like Hildegard von Bingen and Paracelsus offered new insights into plant-based remedies (Newman, 1985; Ball, 2006). The Renaissance period further spurred interest in botany and medicinal plants, leading to detailed herbals that cataloged plant species and their uses (Wachtel-Galor & Benzie, 2011).

In the Americas, the interaction between Indigenous knowledge and European settlers resulted in an enriched pharmacopeia. For example, the discovery of quinine from the bark of the cinchona tree by South American Indigenous peoples offered a breakthrough treatment for malaria. Such exchanges showcased the evolving nature of herbal practices, which adapted and expanded through cultural intersections and scientific advancements (World Health Organization, 2023).

Integration With Modern Medicine

Today, herbal medicine is increasingly integrated with modern medical practices, hence forming part of holistic healthcare approaches. In countries like China and India, traditional practices are formally incorporated into the healthcare system. For instance, the People's Republic of China mandates some formal training in TCM for its modern medicine practitioners, ensuring they are knowledgeable about suitable herbal approaches (Zhang et al., 2011).

In many Western countries, there is an increasing acknowledgment of the advantages of combining herbal treatments with standard medical practices. Institutions such as the U.S. National Institutes of Health (NIH) and the Australian National Institute of Complementary Medicine (NICM) actively endorse research on the effectiveness and safety of herbal medicines. This fusion has sparked advancements in managing ailments like chronic pain, where natural options like turmeric and ginger are utilized alongside traditional painkillers to improve patient results (Zhang et al., 2011).

The increasing use of technologies such as artificial intelligence (AI) and functional magnetic resonance imaging (fMRI) furthers our understanding of how traditional practices work. AI helps researchers analyze large sets of data from traditional medical knowledge, thereby identifying patterns and potential new treatments. fMRI has enabled the study of brain activity during practices like yoga and meditation, showing measurable relaxation responses that validate these ancient methods (World Health Organization, 2023).

Herbal Medicine Today

More and more people around the globe are turning to herbal medicine as a natural choice instead of prescription drugs. In many poorer nations, it is often the go-to option for health care because it's easy to find and does not cost much. The World Health Organization (WHO) states that up to 80% of people in Africa depend on herbal remedies for their basic health needs. This shows just how vital traditional healing practices are in places where modern hospitals and clinics might not be readily available (2023).

In developed nations, the popularity of herbal medicine is growing among those looking to complement conventional treatments for ailments such as anxiety, sleep disorders, and digestive issues. The global market for herbal supplements is expanding, with products like valerian root for sleep or peppermint oil for irritable bowel syndrome becoming household names (Wachtel-Galor & Benzie, 2011).

There is a growing push to set clear rules and regulations for herbal medicine to make sure products are safe and of high quality. Having solid guidelines for how these products are made and how to report any negative effects is key to keeping consumers confident in herbal remedies. Additionally, studying how these herbs work in our bodies, including their interactions with other drugs, helps lay down a scientific foundation for using them effectively (Zhang et al., 2011).

Furthermore, the integration of herbal medicine into educational curricula and clinical practice guidelines highlights its accepted role in modern healthcare. Medical schools are now offering courses in integrative medicine, combining conventional and alternative treatments to give future healthcare providers a more comprehensive toolkit (Zick et al., 2009).

Key Concepts in Herbal Healing

To truly appreciate herbal medicine, it is important to start with some basic ideas that form the core of this age-old practice. Herbal healing goes beyond just addressing symptoms; it embraces a complete view of health and well-being. Here, we will explore fundamental concepts like treating the whole person, understanding how herbs interact with our bodies, how different ingredients work together, and why it's crucial to tailor remedies to each individual's needs.

Firstly, let's explore the holistic approach. Unlike conventional medicine, which often focuses on treating isolated symptoms, herbal medicine considers the whole person. This perspective means that an herbalist looks at the body, mind, and spirit as interconnected parts of an individual's health. For instance, if someone presents with a headache, an herbalist might consider their stress levels, diet, sleep patterns, and emotional state rather than simply prescribing a remedy to alleviate the pain (Zick et al., 2009). This comprehensive view aims to address the root causes of health issues, promoting overall well-being and balance.

The Concept of the Energetics of Herbs

Next up is the concept of the energetics of herbs. In herbalism, herbs are not just categorized by their chemical constituents but also by their energetic qualities. These qualities can include warming, cooling, drying, or moistening effects. For example, ginger is considered a warming herb, which means it's often used to treat conditions like cold extremities or slow digestion, where warmth is needed. On the other hand, peppermint is cooling and might be used to soothe hot conditions like fever or inflammation. Understanding these energetic properties helps practitioners select the most appropriate herbs for each individual's unique constitution and health needs (Wachtel-Galor & Benzie, 2011).

Synergy of Ingredients

Moving on to the synergy of ingredients, this principle emphasizes how combining different herbs can enhance their overall effectiveness. In herbal medicine, it is common to create blends or formulas that work together in harmony. Each herb in a formula can support the others, creating a balanced and more potent remedy. For example, a digestive blend might include a warming herb like ginger to stimulate digestion, a bitter herb like dandelion to support liver function, and a calming herb like chamomile to reduce inflammation and soothe the stomach lining. This synergy ensures a more comprehensive approach to healing and can therefore improve the efficacy of the treatment (Zick et al., 2009).

Individualization

Lastly, one of the most critical aspects of herbal medicine is individualization. Tailoring herbal remedies to suit individual needs is paramount in this practice. Everybody is different, and what works for one person might not necessarily work for another. An herbalist considers various factors such as age, gender, genetic background, lifestyle, and specific health conditions when recommending treatments. This personalized approach ensures that the remedies are more effective and aligned with the person's unique health profile. For instance, while a general immune-boosting herb like echinacea might benefit many, it may need to be paired with other herbs or adjusted in dosage to suit the specific constitution and needs of an elderly person versus a young adult (Zhang et al., 2011).

To provide some guidelines for individualization, there are a few key points you will want to take into consideration:

- **Personal Health History**: Understand the individual's past health issues, ongoing concerns, and any medications they may be taking. This information helps avoid contraindications and ensures the chosen herbs complement their overall health plan.

- **Constitutional Type**: Determine the person's constitutional type according to traditional systems like Ayurveda or Traditional Chinese Medicine (TCM). This assessment helps identify the most suitable herbs for their body type and current state of health.

- **Lifestyle and Environment**: Consider the individual's daily habits, diet, stress levels, and environmental factors. A remedy tailored to someone living in a cold climate with a high-stress job might differ from one for a person in a warm, relaxed environment.

- **Monitoring and Adjustments**: Herbal treatments should be monitored regularly, and adjustments made as needed. The body's response to herbs can change over time, and ongoing evaluation ensures the treatment remains effective and safe.

- **Patient Engagement**: Encourage individuals to participate actively in their healing process. Educate them about the herbs they are using, their benefits, and any potential side effects. This involvement fosters a deeper connection to their health journey and empowers them to make informed decisions.

By integrating these guidelines, herbalists can create highly personalized treatment plans that respect the unique dynamics of each person's health and lifestyle, optimizing the effectiveness of herbal medicine.

Benefits of Herbal Remedies

One of the central reasons people choose herbal remedies is how natural and easily accessible they are. Unlike some medications that need a doctor's prescription, you can grow a lot of herbs right in your backyard or grab them at health food shops and farmers' markets without any fuss. This ease of access is why herbal remedies appeal to people who want to take charge of their health. Tending to your own medicinal plants, like chamomile, lavender, or peppermint, can also make you feel empowered about your wellness choices. And for those who can't cultivate their own, buying herbs remains a simpler and cheaper option than dealing with the complexities of conventional medicine.

Affordability

Moreover, the affordability of herbal remedies cannot be overstated. Prescription drugs can be prohibitively expensive, particularly for those without insurance. In contrast, herbal treatments can often be a fraction of the cost, making them more accessible to a broader range of people.

The economic advantage of using herbs is particularly crucial for individuals in low-income households or in regions where healthcare options are limited. By reducing the financial burden associated with maintaining health, herbal remedies offer a viable alternative to conventional medicine.

Fewer Side Effects

Another significant benefit of herbal remedies is that they typically have fewer side effects compared to synthetic medications. Many prescription drugs come with a long list of potential adverse effects that can sometimes be severe and even life-threatening. On the other hand, herbs, when used correctly, tend to be gentler on the body. According to a study, a considerable percentage of adults in the United States experience adverse side effects from prescription medications (*What Are the Benefits of Herbal Medicine?* 2022). Herbs such as ginger and turmeric are known for their anti-inflammatory properties and are less likely to cause the gastrointestinal distress that some over-the-counter anti-inflammatory drugs might induce. This reduced risk of side effects is especially important for those who may already be dealing with multiple health conditions and need to avoid additional complications from their treatments.

Promoting Preventive Care

Herbal remedies are key to taking care of our health before problems arise. Instead of waiting to get sick, adding herbs to our daily routine can help keep us feel good and stop diseases before they start. For instance, herbs such as echinacea and elderberry are famous for giving our immune system a boost. Using these herbs regularly can strengthen the defenses of our body, making us less likely to catch a cold or the flu. Likewise, adaptogenic herbs like ashwagandha and rhodiola support us in handling stress better, lowering the chances of stress-related illnesses. This way of thinking fits perfectly with holistic health, which focuses on keeping our body in harmony instead of just treating issues as they come up.

Cultural and Personal Connection to Nature and Individual Health

Using herbs will aid us as we aim to deeply connect to nature and our well-being. Herbal medicine is part of the cultural design worldwide, like in Traditional Chinese Medicine and Ayurveda. When we explore these traditions, we tap into our cultural heritage and the wisdom of those who came before us. For many people, working with herbs goes beyond just physical health, for it is also about nurturing our spiritual and emotional growth. The process of preparing and using herbal remedies can feel like a meditative practice, fostering mindfulness and a greater appreciation for the beauty of the natural world. This holistic approach looks after not only our bodies but also supports our mental and emotional health.

By now, you should feel a little more at ease and acquainted with the concept of herbal remedies as a topic, as you have been given some historical insights that highlight the enduring importance of herbal medicine across different societies and its continued relevance today. The key focus, however, was for you to begin understanding the fundamental concepts of herbal medicine, such as its holistic approach, the energetic properties of herbs, the combination of different ingredients for enhanced effectiveness, and the tailored approach for each individual. These elements set herbal medicine apart from conventional treatments by promoting a personalized and harmonious method of achieving health.

As this chapter has laid the groundwork for understanding the core principles of herbal medicine, this foundational knowledge in hand allows you to embark on your exploration of herbal medicine. Perhaps starting with the coming chapter will guide you through the practical steps you need to take to begin incorporating these natural remedies into your daily life and help you create a personalized approach to health and well-being.

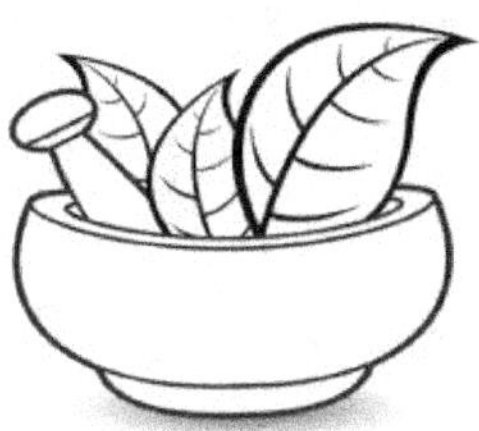

CHAPTER 2

Starting Your Herbal Journey

Starting your herbal adventure begins with getting a better understanding of the key tools and insights that will help you make the most of these natural wonders, which will allow you to effectively prepare your herbs. By gathering some basic items, like a mortar and pestle for grinding, an infuser for steeping, and measuring spoons to get your portions just right, you will be prepared enough to dive deep into the world of herbal preparations. These simple yet crucial tools will not only make it easier to create your herbal remedies but will also help you ensure that each preparation is consistent and works effectively.

While this chapter serves as an exploration of the variety of tools available—both essential and advanced—it will aid you as you venture deeper into the magical, unknown world of herbalism. It is a relatively short, nevertheless sweet, chapter that will examine the importance of proper cleaning and maintenance to extend the lifespan and efficacy of your tools, but also provide insights into setting up an organized and efficient workspace, thus ensuring you have everything you need at your fingertips.

Essential Tools for Herbal Preparation

When beginning your journey into herbal remedies, having the right tools is crucial for efficient preparation and effective use. Understanding the basic equipment and advanced tools available will lay a strong foundation for your practice.

The Necessities

Let us begin by exploring the most essential tools for any herbal enthusiast: the mortar and pestle; indispensable for crushing and grinding herbs to release their active ingredients. This tool is not just an old-fashioned piece; it plays a vital role in preparing herbs effectively. The mortar is a bowl, usually made from a sturdy material like stone, while the pestle is a heavy stick used for grinding. Together, they create a powerful combination that can turn whole herbs into fine powders or crush loose leaves into a usable form.

Using a mortar and pestle is straightforward, and it allows you to release the active ingredients in herbs. When you crush or grind herbs, you help to break down their cell walls. This process makes it easier for the body to access the beneficial compounds contained in them. Moreover, the mortar and pestle maintain the natural properties of the herbs. Many modern tools, like blenders, can heat the ingredients through friction. This heat can destroy some of the delicate properties of herbs. However, with the mortar and pestle, you can work slowly and gently, keeping the herbs in their natural state. This method reflects traditional practices that have been followed for centuries, showcasing the effectiveness of ancient techniques in crafting herbal remedies.

Choosing the Right Mortar and Pestle

When selecting a mortar and pestle, there are several factors to consider. The size of the tools is essential. If you plan to work with larger quantities of herbs, a bigger mortar will serve you well. Likewise, if you focus on single servings or small batches, a smaller version might be more practical. Consider the materials too. Stone or ceramic options are durable and provide a stable surface for grinding. Wooden mortar and pestles can be lighter but might not grind as effectively as stone ones.

Additional Essential Tools

An infuser, which is often used for brewing herbal teas, allows the herbs to steep properly and release their beneficial compounds into hot water and is therefore yet another rather crucial tool, even for the beginner. An infuser is a helpful tool for anyone who enjoys herbal teas. This simple device allows you to brew your favorite herbs effectively. When you place the herbs inside the infuser and submerge them in hot water, it creates an environment where the herbs can steep properly. Steeping is crucial because it enables the herbs to release their beneficial compounds into the water. This means that you get all the good stuff from the herbs, like vitamins and antioxidants, which can have positive effects on your health.

Using an infuser doesn't have to be complicated. For beginners, it's a straightforward way to start exploring the world of herbal teas. You can find different types of infusers made from various materials, including stainless steel, silicone, and even fabric. Each material has its pros and cons. For example, stainless steel is durable and easy to clean, while silicone is flexible and can be squeezed to help release flavors faster. Choose the one that suits your personal preferences.

In addition to an infuser, having measuring spoons is very important when preparing herbal teas, or for achieving precise dosage when preparing your remedies. Accurate measurements help ensure that you use the right amount of each herb, and you can thereby maintain consistency in your preparations. This means that if you find a blend that you like, you can replicate it easily time after time.

Next Level

For those looking to take their herbal practice to the next level, optional advanced tools can significantly enhance your capabilities. Dehydrators are excellent for drying herbs quickly and efficiently, retaining their potency and extending their shelf life. Dried herbs are easier to store and can be used in various formulations from teas to tinctures.

Herbal presses, another advanced tool, are perfect for making herbal extracts and tinctures. These presses help you extract every drop of liquid from your herbs, ensuring maximum efficacy and minimizing waste. Advanced tools, while not necessary for beginners, can open up new possibilities and allow for more sophisticated herbal preparations.

Cleaning and Maintenance

Proper cleaning and maintenance of your herbal equipment is also vital to ensure longevity and effectiveness. Always wash your tools thoroughly after each use, making sure to remove any residues that could harbor bacteria. Glass jars and bottles should be sterilized by running them through the dishwasher or boiled in water. They must be completely dry before use to prevent moisture-induced spoilage (*How to Make Infused Oil*, 2010). Mortar and pestle should be rinsed and dried immediately to prevent herb particles from adhering. For infusers and measuring spoons, a simple rinse with warm, soapy water followed by thorough drying will suffice. Regular maintenance not only enhances the lifespan of your equipment but also ensures that your herbal remedies remain safe to use.

Your Workspace

Setting up a dedicated workspace for herbal preparation can greatly improve your efficiency and enjoyment. Begin by choosing a spot in your home where you can keep all your tools and materials organized and within reach. A sunny windowsill or a well-lit counter space is ideal for this purpose, providing ample light and ventilation. Arrange your equipment methodically, with frequently used items like the mortar and pestle, infuser, and measuring spoons placed conveniently at hand. Personalize your workspace with containers for different herbs, labeled clearly for easy identification. Keeping your workspace clean and orderly will make your herbal practices more enjoyable and less daunting.

Reliable Sources for Herbal Education

It is extremely important that you rely on well-vetted sources of information as you begin your herbal journey, for accurate and reliable knowledge is the cornerstone of successfully incorporating herbal remedies into your health practices. This section will serve as a guide through various reputable sources where you can gather valuable insights about herbs.

Books and Literature

Books remain one of the most reliable resources for herbal education. Not all books are created equal, so it is crucial to access a curated list of recommended readings from reputable authors and publishers. Start with titles that are frequently cited in the herbal community. For example, *The Herbal Medicine-Maker's Handbook* (Green, 2002) and *Rosemary Gladstar's Medicinal Herbs: A Beginner's Guide* (2012) are highly respected in the field. These texts not only provide comprehensive knowledge but also include practical recipes and methods for preparing herbal remedies. When selecting books, look for those written by trained herbalists or those with academic backgrounds in botany or pharmacology to ensure that the information is credible.

Online Courses and Workshops

With the rise of digital learning, numerous online courses and workshops are available to those interested in herbalism. These resources offer flexibility and accessibility, allowing you to learn at your own pace. Renowned institutions often offer these courses, such as the Chestnut School of Herbal Medicine, which provides programs ranging from herbal immersion to foraging courses (Harder, 2019). Massive Open Online Courses (MOOCs) like those found on Coursera or Udemy also offer introductory courses on herbalism. These platforms usually feature experienced instructors who bring a wealth of knowledge and practical experience to their teachings. Participating in workshops allows for hands-on learning and interaction with experts, providing you with deeper insights into the practical aspects of herbalism.

Herbalist Communities and Organizations

Connecting with experienced herbalists and joining established communities can also significantly enhance your learning experience. Local and national organizations often serve as hubs for networking, mentorship, and educational events. Look for groups such as the American Herbalists Guild, which offers resources, forums, and listings of certified practitioners. Being part of these communities exposes you to a wealth of collective knowledge and experience, enabling you to learn from others' successes and challenges. Also, many herbalist communities organize events like herb walks, markets, and conferences, providing opportunities for immersive learning and real-world application of herbal practices.

Podcasts and Blogs

In the digital age, podcasts and blogs have emerged as valuable tools for learning about herbalism. These mediums offer a convenient way to consume information, whether you're commuting, exercising, or relaxing at home. However, it's crucial to assess the credibility of these resources. Reputable podcasts like *Natural MD Radio* by Dr. Aviva Romm and *Real Herbalism Radio* hosted by Candace Hunter and Sue Sierralupé provide insightful discussions on a range of topics from women's health to medicinal mushrooms. Similarly, well-established blogs like "The Herbal Academy" and "LearningHerbs" curate content that combines traditional wisdom with modern science (*Herbal Academy*, 2015; *HerbMentor*, n.d.). When exploring these digital resources, consider the qualifications of the author and cross-reference their information with more formal publications to ensure accuracy.

Creating Your First Herbal Toolkit

Starting your herbal journey can be an exciting and enriching experience. To ensure you begin on the right foot, it is crucial to assemble a well-rounded collection of essential herbs and tools for practical use. This section will guide you through choosing beginner-friendly herbs, proper storage solutions, simple herbal recipes, and the importance of regularly reassessing your herbal toolkit.

Choosing Essential Herbs

When starting with herbal remedies, selecting the right herbs is key. Beginner-friendly herbs are those that are easy to find, versatile in their uses, and generally safe. Consider local availability when making your choices—herbs that grow well in your region are often fresher and more affordable. Some common beginner herbs include:

- **Chamomile**: Known for its calming properties, chamomile can be used to make soothing teas that aid in sleep and digestion.

- **Peppermint**: Versatile and refreshing, peppermint helps with digestive issues and can be used in teas, oils, and even bath soaks.

- **Lavender**: With its relaxing scent, lavender is great for stress relief and skin care, often used in baths and homemade lotions.

- **Echinacea**: Popular during cold and flu season, echinacea is believed to support the immune system.

- **Lemon Balm**: Mild and lemon-scented, this herb helps alleviate anxiety and can be used in teas or as a flavorful addition to salads.

Personal health goals should also guide your herb selection. If you are looking to improve digestion, consider herbs like ginger and fennel. For stress relief, herbs like valerian and passionflower may be beneficial.

Storage Solutions

Proper storage is essential to maintain the freshness and potency of your herbs. Fresh herbs can lose their medicinal qualities if not stored correctly. Here are some tips to ensure your herbs stay effective:

- **Drying**: Air-drying is a popular method for preserving herbs. Hang small bunches upside down in a cool, dark place with good air circulation. Once dried, store the herbs in airtight containers away from direct sunlight.

- **Containers**: Use glass jars with tight-fitting lids to keep out moisture and pests. Clear jars allow you to see the contents but should be stored in a dark cupboard to protect from light.

- **Labeling**: Clearly label each container with the name of the herb and the date it was stored. This practice helps you keep track of freshness and ensures you're using the right herb for your needs.

- **Freezing**: Some herbs, such as basil and parsley, maintain their flavor better when frozen. Chop the herbs and place them in ice cube trays with water or olive oil, then transfer the frozen cubes to labeled freezer bags.

Herbal Recipes for Beginners

Confidence in using herbs grows with practice. Starting with simple recipes can help build your skills and inspire creativity. Here are a few easy-to-make herbal recipes:

- **Simple Herbal Tea Blend**: Combine equal parts chamomile, peppermint, and lemon balm. Steep one teaspoon of the blend in hot water for 5–10 minutes. This tea is calming and aids digestion.

- **Lavender Bath Soak**: Mix one cup of Epsom salts with two tablespoons of dried lavender flowers. Add a few drops of lavender essential oil for extra fragrance. Add the mixture to your bathwater to promote relaxation and soothe sore muscles.

- **Peppermint Salve**: Melt one cup of coconut oil and mix in one-quarter cup of dried peppermint leaves. Let the mixture cool and solidify before applying it to sore muscles or dry skin.

These simple recipes encourage experimentation and will help you get more comfortable with incorporating herbs into your daily routine.

Regular Reassessment of the Toolkit

As you gain knowledge and experience, it is important to periodically reassess and update your herbal toolkit. Regular reassessment ensures your collection remains relevant to your evolving needs and interests. Here are some guidelines for maintaining an efficient herbal toolkit:

- **Seasonal Updates**: Different herbs may be more effective or available during certain seasons. In spring and summer, focus on fresh, cooling herbs; in fall and winter, turn to warm, immune-boosting herbs.

- **Learning New Techniques**: As you explore herbalism, you might discover new preparation methods, such as tinctures or poultices. Incorporate these techniques into your toolkit to expand your range of remedies.

- **Evaluating Effectiveness**: Reflect on which herbs and recipes have been most beneficial for you. Keep notes on your experiences and adjust your toolkit based on what works best.

- **Discarding Old Herbs**: Over time, herbs can lose their potency. Regularly check the freshness of your stored herbs and discard any that have lost their color, aroma, or effectiveness.

By taking these steps, you will ensure your herbal toolkit grows and improves alongside your understanding of herbal remedies.

Having finished this chapter, you are now equipped with the foundational knowledge necessary to begin exploring herbal remedies a bit on your own. After having invested in proper tools, organized a workspace, and perhaps created a routine of how to clean and maintain your tools, you will most likely want to dig into the enticing world of herbal remedies. And please, do dive into it headfirst. However, make sure to tune into this next chapter, in which we will explore some of the most commonly used herbs and their applications, thus guiding you in choosing the best herbs to suit your health and wellness goals. This journey into the diverse world of herbs will expand your understanding and appreciation of these powerful natural allies.

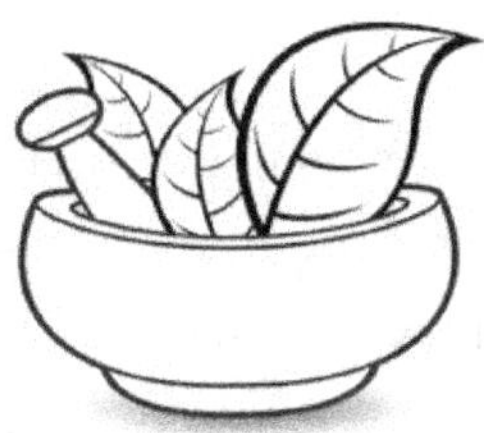

CHAPTER 3

Popular Herbs and Their Uses

Getting to know the must-have herbs for beginners is a rather fundamental part of diving into the world and the art of healing plants and herbalism in general. In this chapter, we will take a closer look at well-loved herbs, while also offering you a friendly guide to their benefits. Each of these herbs comes with its own unique and special qualities that can help with different health issues, thus making them essential, even if you are just starting with herbal remedies. Whether you are looking for stress relief, to get better sleep, to digest your food more easily, or to strengthen your immune system, these versatile herbs all have something valuable to contribute to your journey toward wellness.

Top Herbs for Beginners

As you start your adventure of herbalism, it can feel both thrilling and fulfilling. For newcomers and beginners, understanding the most common and adaptable herbs is crucial for establishing a base in natural healing. Herbs have been utilized for thousands of years to promote health and wellness and have provided a mild yet powerful method for tackling various issues and improving overall health. This section showcases the ten key herbs that are ideal for those new to herbalism. Each herb is chosen for its simplicity, accessibility, and wide array of uses, ensuring a seamless introduction to the world of herbal remedies.

Lavender

Lavender is well-known for its calming effects. This lovely-smelling plant is often used to help reduce stress and improve sleep. The therapeutic, soothing scent of lavender creates a peaceful atmosphere, which is why it is a favorite in aromatherapy. Adding lavender to your daily routine—whether through essential oils, teas, or by enjoying a lavender-infused bath—can really boost your relaxation. Research has found that lavender not only helps you get better sleep but also lifts your mood and eases anxiety. Plus, the benefits of lavender go beyond mental wellness, for it also has anti-inflammatory and antiseptic traits that can be helpful for minor burns, insect bites, and skin irritations (Curtis, 2024).

Peppermint

Peppermint is a remarkably adaptable herb, its crisp, refreshing aroma doing more than delighting the senses—it effectively alleviates digestive problems like indigestion and bloating. The menthol present in peppermint has a calming effect on the muscles in the gastrointestinal tract, providing relief from spasms and discomfort. Sipping on peppermint tea is a popular remedy for soothing stomach issues while offering a cool, revitalizing experience. Moreover, the antiviral and antibacterial qualities of the peppermint make it useful for combating colds and respiratory ailments. Inhaling steam infused with peppermint can help clear nasal passages, thereby making breathing more comfortable during congestion (Thomas, 2020).

Chamomile

Chamomile, a herb often linked to tranquility and better sleep, is both gentle and effective. This plant, resembling a daisy, is celebrated for its anti-inflammatory and antispasmodic benefits, thus, similar to peppermint, making it a great choice for calming an upset stomach and easing muscle cramps. Many enjoy chamomile tea before bed for its subtle sedative qualities that generally help you fall asleep faster and enhance overall sleep quality. In addition to its relaxing attributes, chamomile is also beneficial for skin health. When used topically, it can address ailments like eczema and dermatitis as the anti-inflammatory agents in chamomile work to diminish redness and irritation, thereby also leading to a smoother, healthier complexion (Curtis, 2024; Ruggeri, 2018; Thomas, 2020).

Echinacea

Echinacea is renowned for its ability to enhance immune function, with it being especially beneficial during cold and flu season, as this herb can reduce both the length and intensity of symptoms. By boosting the activity of white blood cells, echinacea strengthens the defenses of the body against infections. It is available in several forms, such as herbal teas, capsules, and tinctures. Furthermore, echinacea is not solely an internal remedy; it can be directly applied to minor wounds to help prevent infection and promote faster healing. This versatile herb has become a staple in many homes as it is cherished for its powerful impact on health and immunity (Curtis, 2024; Ruggeri, 2018; Thomas, 2020).

Basil

Basil is a popular culinary herb treasured for its delightful sweet and slightly peppery fragrance, which makes it a staple in both kitchens and among those creating natural remedies. This herb is rich in essential oils that possess anti-inflammatory and antibacterial effects, making it a superb ally for bolstering the immune system. Additionally, basil is recognized for its ability to aid digestion, often used to craft soothing teas that alleviate discomfort from indigestion and bloating. Furthermore, its potent antioxidant qualities shield the body against oxidative stress, playing a vital role in maintaining overall well-being (Curtis, 2024).

Lemon Balm

Lemon balm is an aromatic herb appreciated mainly for its refreshing lemon fragrance yet recognized for its soothing and uplifting properties. It is frequently utilized to ease feelings of anxiety and tension, as it fosters a sense of tranquility and emotional harmony. You can savor lemon balm as a comforting tea or incorporate it into your bath for a rejuvenating experience. Not to mention the fact that it possesses antiviral characteristics and may therefore bolster the immune system during periods of illness such as when having a cold or the flu (Thomas, 2020).

Rosemary

Rosemary, a fragrant herb known for its robust, piney aroma, is often featured in various culinary creations. Its stimulating qualities can boost memory and focus and therefore make it a perfect ally for mental clarity. Additionally, rosemary boasts anti-inflammatory and antioxidant properties that promote immune health and improve circulation. Whether enjoyed as a soothing tea or used in essential oil form, or perhaps to spice up your lamb dish, rosemary revitalizes both mind and body as it enhances your cognitive abilities and overall vitality (Ruggeri, 2018).

Turmeric

Turmeric is a striking yellow spice, well-known among herbalists and common folk alike, for its powerful anti-inflammatory and antioxidant characteristics. Its active component, curcumin, is the focus of numerous studies highlighting its effectiveness in alleviating inflammation and promoting joint well-being (Agrawal & Goel, 2016; Hewlings & Kalman, 2017; Daily et al., 2016). You can enjoy turmeric in several ways, such as steeping it in teas, taking it in capsule form, or adding it to your favorite recipes for a delightful twist. The benefits of turmeric also include boosting digestive health and aiding liver function by facilitating detoxification. Consistently incorporating turmeric into your diet may lower the likelihood of chronic illnesses, attributed to its capacity to combat free radicals and strengthen the body's antioxidant system (Curtis, 2024; Ruggeri, 2018).

Ginger

Ginger is a flavorful and invigorating root that comes with a multitude of health benefits, especially its ability to combat nausea. It effectively addresses issues like motion sickness, pregnancy-related nausea (although one should be a bit careful with ginger during pregnancy), and digestive unease. Ginger also has anti-inflammatory and antioxidant properties which enhance joint health and mitigate swelling. Whether enjoyed as a soothing tea, incorporated into dishes, or utilized in essential oils, ginger works to rejuvenate the body and foster overall wellness (Curtis, 2024; Ruggeri, 2018).

Thyme

Thyme is a versatile herb praised for its potent antiseptic and antimicrobial qualities. It's a popular choice for enhancing respiratory wellness, making it a fantastic solution for alleviating coughs and colds. Thyme can be prepared as a tea or incorporated into steam inhalation to relieve congestion and promote easier breathing. Its carminative properties also aid digestion, reducing gas and bloating. With such a wide array of uses, thyme is definitely a must-have herb for anyone who is just starting in herbal remedies (Indigo Herbs, 2014; Ruggeri, 2018).

Ginseng

Lastly, the powerful adaptogenic herb ginseng is celebrated mainly for its ability to enhance energy, reduce stress, and improve overall well-being. Known for its rejuvenating properties, ginseng helps the body adapt to physical and mental stressors, making it a popular choice for boosting endurance and mental performance. It is also often used to support immune function and increase vitality, thanks to its antioxidant and anti-inflammatory effects. Ginseng can be consumed as a tea, in capsules, or as a supplement to enhance cognitive function and combat fatigue (Curtis, 2024; Ruggeri, 2018). It has also been studied for its potential to lower blood sugar levels and improve circulation, contributing to a healthier metabolic profile (Shishtar et al., 2014).

Properties and Benefits of the Herbs

Antioxidant

Antioxidant-rich herbs like rosemary, basil, ginger, and ginseng play a crucial role in maintaining our health by combating oxidative stress, which occurs when there is an imbalance between free radicals and antioxidants in the body. Free radicals are unstable molecules that can damage cells, leading to chronic diseases and aging. Rosemary, for example, is known for its robust flavor and aroma and contains compounds such as carnosic acid and rosmarinic acid that neutralize these harmful molecules. Hence, by incorporating rosemary, basil, ginger, and ginseng into your diet, either through culinary use or herbal teas, you can help protect your body from oxidative damage (Curtis, 2024; Gladstar, 2012; Ruggeri, 2018).

Anti-inflammatory

Inflammation is a natural response of the immune system, but chronic inflammation can lead to various health issues, including arthritis, heart disease, and cancer. The active compound in turmeric, curcumin, has, as previously stated, been extensively studied for its ability to reduce inflammation at the molecular level (Agrawal & Goel, 2016; Hewlings & Kalman, 2017; Daily et al., 2016). Curcumin inhibits the activity of inflammatory enzymes and cytokines, providing relief from conditions like joint pain and swelling. Including turmeric in your diet, whether through cooking or supplements, can help manage inflammation and support long-term health.

Immune Boosting

Thyme is a great example of a herb that significantly boosts the immune system of your body. It contains thymol, an antiseptic compound that combats bacteria and viruses. Regular consumption of thyme, whether in the form of fresh leaves, dried herb, or essential oil, can help prevent respiratory infections and by extension also improve your overall immune function. Other herbs that also greatly enhance your immune system and should be incorporated into your daily intake if you are suffering from a weak immune system, are echinacea, basil, rosemary, and ginseng (Curtis, 2024).

Cognitive Function

On the topic of ginseng, even though great for boosting your immune system, it is mostly famous for its ability to enhance cognitive function and reduce fatigue. Ginseng contains ginsenosides, which have neuroprotective effects and therefore improve mental performance. These compounds help increase the release of acetylcholine, a neurotransmitter involved in learning and memory. This herb also supports energy levels by enhancing physical stamina and reducing feelings of exhaustion. Regular use of ginseng, but also rosemary for similar qualities, can contribute to more mental clarity and sustained energy throughout the day (Ruggeri, 2018).

Incorporation

Beyond merely understanding the various characteristics of these mentioned beginner herbs, you also need to understand their practical applications and how to incorporate them into daily life. For instance, while rosemary can be used in cooking to season meats, vegetables, and soups, its essential oil can be diffused for aromatherapy benefits which would promote concentration and relieve stress. Turmeric is versatile and can be added to curries and smoothies or made into a soothing golden milk drink, while thyme is excellent for seasoning dishes, making herbal teas, or even gargling with (as a thyme infusion) to alleviate sore throats.

Other than their culinary uses, these herbs can also be utilized in various forms such as capsules, extracts, and essential oils, with each of these providing their own unique benefits. Rosemary essential oil, for example, can be massaged into the scalp to stimulate hair growth and improve circulation. Turmeric supplements in the form of capsules or tablets offer a concentrated dose of curcumin for those needing targeted anti-inflammatory support. Similarly, thyme essential oil can be diluted and applied topically to treat skin infections and inflammation.

Furthermore, creating a holistic approach to using these herbs involves combining them with other lifestyle practices. For instance, pairing a diet rich in antioxidant herbs like rosemary with regular exercise and adequate sleep can amplify the benefits and create a balanced, healthy lifestyle. Incorporating turmeric into an anti-inflammatory diet that reduces processed foods and sugars can further support its effects on managing inflammation. Using thyme alongside other immune-boosting practices, such as regular hand washing and stress management techniques, can further enhance their protective roles.

It is also important to recognize the safety and dosage recommendations for these herbs. While generally safe, excessive consumption can lead to adverse effects. For example, high doses of rosemary oil may cause skin irritation, and large amounts of turmeric can upset the stomach. Consulting with a healthcare provider or a qualified herbalist before starting any new herbal regimen is advisable, especially for individuals with pre-existing health conditions or those taking medications, or if you feel unsure of your own capacity and knowledge of said herbs. We were all beginners at one point, and rather safe than sorry, so make sure you study the potential effects of these herbs in-depth before indulging in herbalist work, on yourself or for others.

Common Conditions

Nausea and Digestive Issues

Ginger is a potent herb with versatile applications, however, particularly potent when it comes to alleviating nausea and aiding digestive issues. This root has been a staple in traditional medicine for centuries, renowned for its effectiveness in treating various gastrointestinal disturbances. Gingerol, the active compound in ginger, possesses powerful anti-inflammatory and antioxidant properties, which contribute to its therapeutic benefits. For instance, consuming ginger tea or supplements can significantly reduce symptoms of nausea, whether from motion sickness, pregnancy, or chemotherapy. Yet, as previously stated, if you are pregnant, you should consult your midwife and physician before eating ginger, as too much ginger in early pregnancy might come with unwanted and negative side effects. Furthermore, ginger helps stimulate digestion by enhancing bile production, making it an excellent remedy for indigestion, bloating, and constipation.

Other herbs that target nausea and/or digestive issues are for example peppermint and turmeric.

Supporting Digestive Health

Good digestion is essential for feeling our best and keeping our bodies running smoothly. When our digestive system works well, it helps us get the necessary nutrients from what we eat, which supports our energy and overall health. On the other hand, when digestion is off, it can cause problems like tiredness, a run-down immune system, and ongoing stomach issues. By including herbal remedies in our daily lives, we can find natural ways to ease discomfort and boost our digestive health, paving the way for a happier, healthier life.

As mentioned, one herb that stands out for its digestive benefits is peppermint. Peppermint oil is great for easing tummy troubles, especially for those dealing with IBS. Studies show that peppermint capsules can really help with stomach pain, bloating, and gas. This benefit comes from menthol, which relaxes the gut muscles. It also supports bile production, helping with fat digestion. You can enjoy peppermint tea or take capsules as a supplement. Just check with your doctor first to avoid any medication conflicts (Streit, 2019).

Ginger is a remarkable herb beloved for its ability to ease digestion. This amazing root, Zingiber officinale, is cherished around the world for its healing qualities. The compounds gingerols and shogaols help the stomach work more efficiently, which can ease nausea, cramping, and gas. Research shows ginger can effectively tackle nausea from pregnancy, chemotherapy, and even motion sickness. Plus, its anti-inflammatory properties are great for soothing digestive issues. You can enjoy ginger fresh, dried, or as a comforting tea; just boil sliced ginger in water for a delightful drink that supports digestion before or after meals (Huddy, 2024).

Chamomile tea is also great for your stomach! It is famous for soothing nerves and can ease indigestion. Perfect for both kids and those with sensitive stomachs, it relaxes the digestive muscles and therefore helps with gas and discomfort. It might even keep pesky ulcers at bay. Enjoying a cup before bed could really help your digestion and help you unwind, especially considering that it also has calming properties.

Dandelion, often dismissed as just a weed, deserves a closer look even though it was overlooked in the previous list. It offers remarkable health perks, especially for digestion and liver health, acting as a gentle diuretic that aids detoxification. Dandelion boosts overall well-being and is packed with vital nutrients like vitamins A, C, D, B-complex, iron, potassium, and zinc (Huddy, 2024). Enjoy it in tea or toss the greens into your salad for a nutritious touch. Just make sure it's free from pesticides and chemicals!

Respiratory Health

Moving on to respiratory health with thyme and peppermint, but also the not previously mentioned eucalyptus, are invaluable herbs known for their ability to support respiratory function and manage cold symptoms. Thyme contains thymol, a natural antiseptic that helps combat respiratory infections and alleviate coughs and sore throats. Its expectorant properties make it effective in clearing mucus and easing bronchitis symptoms. Meanwhile, eucalyptus is rich in eucalyptol, which has been shown to reduce inflammation and help open up nasal passages, thereby facilitating easier breathing. Inhalation of eucalyptus essential oil or using it in chest rubs can significantly relieve sinus congestion, colds, and even asthma. A combined use of thyme, peppermint, and eucalyptus can be particularly beneficial during cold and flu seasons as it offers a natural alternative to over-the-counter medications.

Anxiety and Stress

Ashwagandha is an adaptogenic herb we have not yet discussed, but it is highly valued for its ability to reduce stress and anxiety. Since it is not as easily accessible everywhere, it fell out of the top list of beginner herbs; however, it is still a potent and highly recommended herb to utilize and get to know. Adaptogens like this herb are unique in that they help the body adapt to stressors and restore balance. Ashwagandha contains compounds called withanolides, which have neuroprotective and anti-anxiety effects. Regular consumption of ashwagandha, either in powder form, capsules, or tea, can help lower cortisol levels—the body's primary stress hormone—thus promoting a sense of calm and well-being. Moreover, it supports overall mental health by improving focus, reducing fatigue, and enhancing overall cognitive function. Ashwagandha's role in mitigating the impact of chronic stress makes it a valuable addition to natural wellness routines. Other herbs that combat anxiety and stress include lavender, basil, and ginseng.

Skincare

We could not go on without at least briefly mentioning skincare, and for skincare, aloe vera and calendula, also not previously mentioned, stand out as exceptional herbs for soothing minor skin irritations. Aloe vera gel, extracted from the plant's leaves, is widely recognized for its cooling and healing properties and is therefore particularly effective in treating burns, including sunburn, also due to its ability to accelerate skin repair. Aloe vera also provides relief from itching and swelling associated with insect bites and other skin conditions. On the other hand, calendula, often used in ointments and creams, boasts anti-inflammatory, antimicrobial, and wound-healing properties. Its application can help soothe rashes, eczema, and diaper rash, making it a gentle yet effective option for sensitive skin. Both aloe vera and calendula can be easily incorporated into daily skincare routines to maintain healthy, resilient skin, but they can be quite tricky to find in their natural form, hence, being left out of the top list above.

Growing and Harvesting Tips

Understanding each herb's sunlight and soil requirements is crucial for ensuring successful growth. Most herbs thrive in well-drained soil with a pH level of 6.0 to 7.0. The amount of sunlight needed varies by herb, but many prefer four to six hours of direct sunlight daily (Marquesen & Kagan, 2021). For instance, rosemary and thyme flourish in full sun, while parsley and cilantro can tolerate partial shade. Before planting, determine what each herb needs and group them accordingly in your garden.

Harvesting Methods

Harvesting your herbs correctly is vital for maximizing their flavor and ensuring they last longer. By regularly trimming stems, you not only promote fresh growth but also keep your plants thriving. When gathering herbs like basil and mint, gently pinch the stems just above a leaf node; for parsley or chives, trim the stems close to the base. The ideal time to harvest is early morning after the dew has evaporated but before the sun gets too hot, as this is when the essential oils are at their most concentrated. Avoid heavy harvesting as the growing season wraps up to help perennial plants build up energy for the colder months (Chadwick, 2021).

Storing

Taking care of your freshly picked herbs is essential for keeping them fresh and full of their wonderful benefits, in other words, it is important that you store them properly. After you have harvested them, gently wash away any dirt and make sure to dry them off completely to avoid any mold. For best results, tuck them away in airtight containers stored in a cool, dark spot. Glass jars with secure lids are perfect for dried herbs. If you have fresh herbs that you will be using soon, you can simply place them in open plastic bags in the refrigerator crisper. Do not forget to label your containers—many dried herbs can look quite similar, and you would not want to mix them up!

Besides drying and keeping herbs, freezing provides a fantastic way to preserve them, particularly for tender ones like basil and cilantro which can lose their essence when dried. Start by washing and chopping your herbs, then place them in ice cube trays with water or olive oil. After they're frozen, just move the cubes to a freezer bag. This technique lets you easily throw in flavorful herbs to your soups, stews, and sauces all year round (Chadwick, 2021).

Pest Management

Using natural methods to keep your herb garden thriving is a wonderful way to avoid harmful chemicals. One lovely approach is companion planting, where you pair specific plants together to keep pests at bay. For instance, if you grow basil near your tomatoes, you will find that it helps keep pesky flies and mosquitoes away. Marigolds have their charm too, as they help lower nematode numbers in the soil. By inviting helpful insects like ladybugs and lacewings into your garden, you can effectively manage aphids and other nuisances, allowing your garden to flourish without any synthetic substances. Embracing these friendly little allies encourages a healthy ecosystem right in your backyard (Chadwick, 2021; Marquesen & Kagan, 2021).

Growing Indoors

For those looking to grow herbs indoors or in containers, it is important to replicate outdoor conditions as closely as possible. As indoor herbs need ample sunlight, you will want to place them near a south or west-facing window. If natural light is insufficient, you may want to consider using grow lights to supplement. Ensure that container-grown herbs have good drainage by using pots with holes and a quality potting mix. Watering indoor herbs can be more challenging than outdoor plants; be careful not to overwater, as root rot can quickly become an issue.

Watering and Soil Fertility

Continuing the topic of water, it is fair to say that once established, many herbs are relatively low maintenance and drought-tolerant, which makes them ideal for busy gardeners. However, during dry periods, consistent watering practices are necessary. Water deeply in the early morning to allow the roots to absorb moisture before the heat of the day causes evaporation. Mulching around the bases of the plants helps retain soil moisture and suppress weeds, which may compete for nutrients and water.

Taking care of the health of the soil is another critical component of growing herbs. While these plants do not need a lot of nutrients, adding a little compost or organic fertilizer can enhance the quality of the soil and supply the right nutrients. Just be careful with fertilizers that are high in nitrogen, since too much can cause lots of leafy growth but not enough of the flavorful oils, which can diminish the taste and healing benefits of your herbs (Marquesen & Kagan, 2021).

Experimentation

If you want to take your gardening journey to the next level, try out various ways to propagate your plants. While you can certainly start many herbs from seeds, some, such as rosemary and sweet bay, thrive better when started from cuttings. Using a mix of perlite and vermiculite is a great way to help those cuttings take root. To keep things cozy for your young plants, you can cover them with plastic to create a humid environment until they settle in. This technique not only improves your gardening know-how but also helps you quickly grow more of your beloved herbs (Chadwick, 2021).

When to Stop

Knowing when to stop harvesting is equally important for perennial herbs, which require time to prepare for colder months. By late summer, discontinue harvesting to allow these plants to store carbohydrates and energy needed to survive the winter. Cutting back too aggressively late in the season can weaken the plants and reduce their chances of overwintering successfully (Chadwick, 2021).

Lastly, engaging in regular garden maintenance, such as weeding and monitoring for signs of disease, keeps your herb garden productive and healthy. Weeds compete for resources and can harbor pests, making it important to remove them promptly. Keep an eye out for common diseases like powdery mildew and rust, which can affect herb plants, and manage them using organic methods such as neem oil or baking soda sprays.

With this chapter having provided an insightful exploration into the world of medicinal herbs, it is now time to transition to the next chapter, where we will explore how to transform these raw, harvested, herbal materials into usable forms such as tinctures, salves, and infusions. You will be provided with step-by-step guidance on preparing and preserving herbs to maintain their potency and efficacy, and in taking part in that guidance, further enriching your herbal practice and deepening your connection to natural healing.

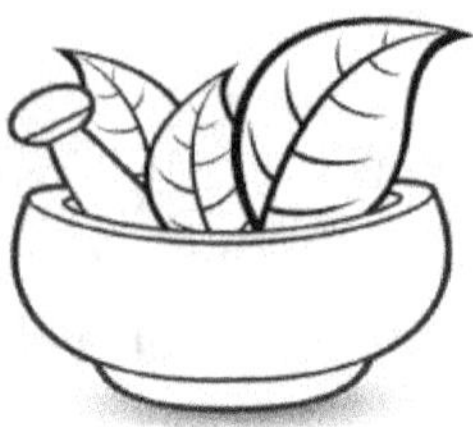

CHAPTER 4

Herbal Preparation Methods

Creating your herbal remedies is a time-honored tradition that is making a comeback as many are turning to nature for their health needs. In this chapter, you will discover key methods for brewing herbal teas, crafting tinctures, and making salves, along with tips on how to store them properly. The abundance of herbs available not only provides countless health benefits—from helping with digestion to improving sleep—but also gives you the chance to take charge of your wellness more naturally. This chapter that guides you through herbal preparation is designed to be a friendly companion for you, helping even the most inexperienced of hearts take confident steps into this rewarding world.

Making Herbal Teas and Infusions

For ages, people have treasured herbal teas, not just for their lovely tastes, but also for the myriad health perks they bring. Different from the usual teas derived from the Camellia sinensis plant, herbal teas are crafted from a mix of herbs, blossoms, seeds, and roots. This variety means there's something for everyone, aligning perfectly with personal health goals and flavor likes. Whether it is aiding digestion, easing stress, promoting restful sleep, or offering a soothing way to stay hydrated, herbal teas have so much to offer. Popular options like chamomile, peppermint, ginger, and hibiscus each come with their unique qualities and advantages.

Steeping Time and Temperature

Crafting a perfect herbal tea or infusion is an art that involves understanding the right steeping times and temperatures to extract maximum benefits while achieving the desired flavor profile. To begin, select your herbs—dried or fresh—and measure about one teaspoon of dried herbs per cup of water. For most herbal infusions, it's crucial to use freshly boiled water. Pour the hot water over the herbs in a pot or directly into a cup. Cover the vessel to prevent the essential oils from escaping with the steam. Generally, steeping times vary between 5 to 15 minutes, depending on the herb's potency and the strength of tea desired. For instance, more delicate herbs like chamomile might need just a short steep of around five minutes, whereas tougher roots like ginger may require the full 15 minutes to release their flavors and nutrients fully (*The health benefits of 3 herbal teas,* 2021). Once the steeping period is up, strain the herbs from the liquid, and your herbal tea is ready to enjoy.

Flavor Enhancing

Elevating the taste of herbal teas can be an enjoyable journey with great rewards. Using natural sweeteners like honey brings a delightful sweetness while offering health advantages, including its natural ability to fight germs. A splash of lemon juice not only lightens the flavor but delivers a refreshing dose of vitamin C, thus boosting the immune-boosting properties of the tea. Adding spices like cinnamon, cardamom, or nutmeg can infuse the brew with a cozy and rich character. Playing around with these ingredients lets you craft a unique blend that perfectly matches your taste and wellness aspirations.

Safety Considerations

When you are getting ready to brew some herbal tea, it is really important to think about safety. Most herbs are fine, but a few can create issues with medications or even trigger unwanted reactions in some folks. Be mindful of allergies—if you are allergic to daisies, for instance, it is best to steer clear of chamomile since they are related. Similarly, if ragweed bothers you, echinacea or dandelion might not be a good fit. It is therefore always smart to chat with your doctor if you have any health concerns or are on any medication. If you are pregnant, definitely check in with your healthcare provider before trying herbs like rosemary, ginger, or turmeric, as they might not be safe for you (Schiller, 2024; *The health benefits of 3 herbal teas*, 2021).

Drinking too much of certain herbal teas can sometimes lead to unpleasant outcomes. Take licorice root tea, for instance. While many love it for its ability to reduce inflammation, it is important not to make it a daily habit for over four weeks, as it might increase blood pressure and decrease potassium levels (*The health benefits of 3 herbal teas*, 2021). Similarly, if you are a fan of rosemary tea, be mindful—overindulging could lead to stomach troubles and other issues. Knowing the right amounts and timeframes for enjoying these teas can help you avoid any potential problems and keep your teatime both safe and delightful (Schiller, 2024).

Preparing Tinctures and Extracts

Herbal tinctures represent one of the most potent forms of herbal medicine, as they are concentrated liquid extracts, typically made by soaking herbs in alcohol to pull out active constituents. The resulting solution captures the essence of the herb in a form that is easy to ingest and absorb into the bloodstream. Tinctures offer extended shelf life, ease of use, and increased potency compared to other preparations like teas or infusions. They are especially beneficial for those who wish to integrate herbal practices into their daily health routines.

Alcohol-Based Tincture

Creating a tincture at home can be an enjoyable and rewarding process, and to make it easier you can follow this step-by-step guide that will walk you through the necessary steps:

1. **Choosing Your Herbs**: Start by selecting high-quality organic dried or fresh herbs. Dried herbs are often preferred as they don't contain excess water that can dilute the tincture. If using fresh herbs, make sure they are clean and free of pesticides.

2. **Materials and Ratios**: You will need a glass jar with a tight-fitting lid, high-proof alcohol (like vodka or brandy), your chosen herbs, and a strainer or cheesecloth. For dried herbs, fill the jar about halfway with the herbs and then cover it completely with alcohol. When using fresh herbs, pack the jar loosely with chopped plant material before covering it with alcohol.

Preparation Steps:

- Place your herbs in the jar and pour in enough alcohol to cover them by at least an inch.

- Seal the jar tightly and store it in a cool, dark place. Shake the jar daily to help the extraction process.

- Allow the mixture to steep for 4–6 weeks, continuing to shake it regularly.

- **Straining and Bottling**: After the steeping period, strain the mixture through a fine-mesh sieve or cheesecloth into another clean container. Squeeze out any remaining liquid from the herbs. Pour the tincture into dark glass bottles to protect it from light.

Non-Alcoholic Tincture

Glycerin offers an excellent alternative for those who prefer non-alcoholic tinctures. Known as glycerites, these are gentler and not as potent as alcohol-based tinctures but are suitable for children and adults who avoid alcohol. Glycerol, derived from vegetables, effectively extracts the active compounds from fresh herbs. When using dried herbs, it's essential to add water to rehydrate them and enhance extraction. The typical ratio for a glycerite is 75% vegetable glycerin and 25% distilled water (Heidi, 2024).

Here is an example of how you can make a herbal glycerite at home:

1. **Ingredients**:
   - Organic herbs (dried or fresh)
   - Organic vegetable glycerin
   - Distilled water (for dried herbs)

2. **Directions for Dried Herbs**:
   - Grind the herbs to increase the surface area.
   - Fill a clean jar halfway with the ground herbs.
   - In a separate jar, mix three parts glycerin with one part distilled water. Shake well to combine.
   - Pour the glycerin-water mixture over the herbs until they are fully covered by one inch.

3. **Directions for Fresh Herbs**:
   - Chop the plant material thoroughly.
   - Fill a clean jar nearly to the top with the chopped herbs.
   - Pour pure vegetable glycerin over the herbs until they are fully covered by one inch.

For both dried and fresh herb preparations, use a long, clean utensil to release any air bubbles. Cap the jar tightly, label it with the contents and the date, and set it aside to macerate for 4–6 weeks. Shake the jar daily and ensure the plant material remains covered. After the maceration period, strain the glycerite through multiple layers of cheesecloth and bottle it in dark glass containers (Heidi, 2024).

Storing Tinctures

To keep your tinctures and glycerites effective and safe, it is essential to store them properly. If you have alcohol-based tinctures, you're in luck—they can stay good for about 4 to 6 years if you treat them right. Make sure to tuck them away in a cool, dark spot, far from the sun's rays and sudden temperature changes. Do not forget to label each bottle with the name of the herb, the ingredient ratios, and when you made them.

Glycerites, on the other hand, have a shorter shelf life of approximately 1–2 years if no alcohol is added. Like tinctures, they should be stored in a cool, dark place. It is essential to keep them out of reach of children and pets, as the sweet taste of glycerin can be tempting.

Incorporating homemade tinctures and glycerites into your routine can significantly enhance your self-care regimen. They are portable, easy to use, and require only small doses due to their concentrated nature. As you gain experience, you may experiment with different herbs and combinations to find what works best for you and your family's needs. Always use herbs responsibly and consider consulting with a healthcare provider if you are new to herbal medicine or if you have any existing health conditions.

Crafting Salves and Balms

Salves and balms are gentle applications rooted in the wisdom of herbal healing, cherished for their ability to comfort, mend, and shield the skin. Crafted from a blend of nurturing oils, healing herbs, and natural beeswax, these remedies provide a holistic alternative to commercial ointments that often contain harsh chemicals. Salves have a richer, firmer texture, while balms are more pliable, thanks to their elevated oil content. Both are wonderful allies for a range of skin issues, including minor cuts, scrapes, insect bites, dry patches, and light burns.

Creating your herbal salves at home is easier than it might seem. By following a straightforward recipe, you can customize the ingredients to address specific needs or preferences. Here is a basic recipe by Dynys (2019) to get you started:

Ingredients:

- 1 1/2 ounces olive oil infused with calendula flowers
- 1 ounce olive oil infused with goldenseal (or more calendula oil)
- 1 ounce olive oil infused with plantain
- 1 tablespoon tamanu oil
- 1/2 ounce beeswax pastilles
- 15 drops of tea tree oil
- 20 drops of lavender essential oil
- 1/8 teaspoon rosemary antioxidants (optional, to lengthen shelf life)

Instructions:

1. **Prepare the Herbal Oils**: Start by infusing your oils with herbs. For a slow infusion method, place dried herbs in a mason jar until it's 1/4 to 1/2 full. Pour olive oil over the herbs until the jar is almost full. Cap the jar, shake it, and let it sit in a cool, dark place for 4 to 6 weeks before straining. This method ensures a potent infusion but requires patience. Alternatively, for a faster method, fill 1/3 to 1/2 of a mason jar with dried herbs and cover with oil. Place the jar in a saucepan filled with a few inches of water and carefully heat on low for 2 to 3 hours. Be sure not to let the oil get too hot, as this can diminish the potency and quality of your infused oil.

2. **Melt the Beeswax**: In a heatproof measuring cup or jar, combine the infused oils, tamanu oil, and beeswax pastilles. Set this into a saucepan with a few inches of water. Heat gently until the beeswax has completely melted, stirring occasionally to ensure everything is well combined.

3. **Add Essential Oils**: Once the mixture is melted and blended, remove it from heat. Add the tea tree oil, lavender essential oil,

and optional rosemary antioxidants to the mixture. Stir well to incorporate the essential oils evenly throughout the salve.

4. **Pour and Cool**: Pour the mixture into small tins or glass jars. Allow them to cool completely before sealing. This step is crucial for the salve to set properly. Once cooled, cap the containers and label them accordingly.

Oil Infusion

Blending oils with herbs is a fundamental practice for crafting powerful herbal salves. This approach helps extract the healing qualities of the herbs into the oil, creating an effective foundation for your salve. Selecting the right herbs is crucial. Many people favor calendula, goldenseal, and plantain due to their soothing and restorative effects. Calendula works wonders for easing irritation, while goldenseal provides antibacterial support, and plantain shines in promoting wound recovery. The infusion method you choose can impact how strong your final product is. Taking your time with a slow infusion at room temperature over a few weeks will result in a rich, potent oil, whereas a quicker, heated infusion can be a practical choice when you're short on time (Visser, 2015).

Storing Oil Infusions

Proper storage of your salves is vital to maintaining their efficacy and extending their shelf life. Store your finished salves in a cool, dark place away from direct sunlight and heat, which can degrade the essential oils and other ingredients. Using amber or cobalt blue glass jars can also help protect the contents from light exposure. It's also important to ensure that the containers you use are clean and dry before pouring the salve into them. Contaminated containers can introduce bacteria or mold, compromising the quality of your salve.

The shelf life of herbal salves can vary depending on the ingredients used and how they are stored. Generally, a well-made salve stored correctly can last up to a year. Adding a natural preservative like rosemary antioxidants can further extend the shelf life. Always check your salves for any changes in smell, color, or texture, which can indicate spoilage. If you notice any off-putting odors or signs of mold, it's best to discard the salve and make a fresh batch.

Drying and Storing Herbs Properly

Drying and storing herbs is a crucial step in preserving their potency and effectiveness, making them ready for use whenever needed. Without proper techniques, however, herbs can lose their beneficial properties or spoil quickly. Freshly harvested herbs, for instance, contain moisture, which, if not adequately removed, can promote mold and bacterial growth. This not only impacts the medicinal qualities of the herb but also renders it unsafe for consumption. Drying removes this moisture, thereby prolonging its shelf life while preserving essential oils, color, and flavor.

Drying Herbs

There are several methods for drying herbs, each suitable for different types of herbs and available resources. One common method is air drying. To air dry, gather a small bunch of herbs and tie their stems together with twine. Hang the bundles upside down in a warm, dark, and well-ventilated area. This technique works best for hearty herbs like rosemary, thyme, and oregano. It generally takes about one to two weeks for the herbs to become dry and brittle.

An alternative to air drying is using a drying screen. Spread the herbs out on a screen suspended over chairs or another structure that allows air to circulate both above and below the screen. Keep the herbs in a dust-free, airy place away from direct sunlight. Herbs with smaller leaves like basil and parsley typically take up to two weeks to dry completely.

For quicker results, a food dehydrator can be used. Preheat the dehydrator to around 100°F (37°C) and arrange the herbs in a single layer on the dehydrator trays. Depending on the type of herb, it may take between one to four hours for them to dry. It's essential to check periodically to avoid over-drying, as this can lead to a loss of potency (Rachel, 2016).

Storing

Once the herbs are fully dried, proper storage techniques are critical to maintain their quality. The key here lies in minimizing exposure to air, light, heat, and moisture. Start by removing the leaves from the stems and storing them loosely in clean glass jars or containers with airtight lids. Glass jars with screw-top lids or metal tins with tight-sealing lids are preferred for their non-reactive nature. Avoid plastic containers as they can introduce unwanted chemicals into the herbs.

Store your containers in a cool, dark place away from direct sunlight and heat sources. A pantry or cupboard works well but ensure it's not near the stove or other appliances that generate heat. For optimal storage conditions, keep the temperature between 50°F (10°C) and 70°F (21°C). Ensure the environment is dry to prevent moisture from compromising the herbs' integrity (*How Long Do Dried Herbs Last?* n.d.).

Labeling

Keeping your herb collection tidy and well-labeled is essential for enjoying it to the fullest. Take a moment to write down the name of each herb along with when you packed it into its jar. This simple act makes finding what you need a breeze, and it allows you to monitor how fresh and potent each herb remains. By storing your herbs in a special cabinet or drawer away from other strong-smelling foods, you help maintain their delightful scents.

Keeping Track

Evaluating how dried herbs hold up over time means checking in on them regularly, focusing on how they look, smell, and their expiration details. A strong fragrance and unique taste are essential signs of how powerful an herb is. If the aroma fades or becomes musty, it's probably time to let it go. Likewise, top-notch dried herbs usually keep a lively color. If they appear notably faded or off-color, it might mean they've lost their effectiveness, hinting that they won't deliver the flavor or health benefits you're hoping for.

Grasping the meaning of expiration and best-by dates is crucial for keeping your herbal stock fresh and effective. Although herbs don't come with a strict expiration date, they typically remain good for about one to three years. Beyond that, you might notice a slow fade in their fragrance and taste. Whole spices and herbs tend to stick around a bit longer than their ground counterparts since they have a smaller exposed surface area. Whole spices can usually keep their strength for around four to five years, while ground spices are at their finest when used within two to four years after buying them.

Keeping track of how long your herbs last is essential to make sure you use them at their best. Take a moment to look over your herb containers regularly for any hints of mold or dampness, as these can affect their safety and usefulness. By following these simple steps, you'll ensure that your dried herbs stay a cherished part of your collection, always available to offer their lovely benefits when you need them most.

As you are now more comfortable with the essential techniques for preparing a variety of herbal remedies, you should also feel empowered to incorporate these practices into your daily routines safely and effectively. By mastering the art of crafting herbal teas, tinctures, and salves, you should now be able to confidently explore natural health solutions tailored to your needs. As we move into the next chapter, we will begin investigating how to best incorporate these herbal preparations into your everyday routines to support your health and wellness. Whether starting the day with a calming herbal tea or using a restorative salve for self-care, these practices can enhance overall vitality and resilience; you just have to figure out how to best utilize them all for your purposes and needs.

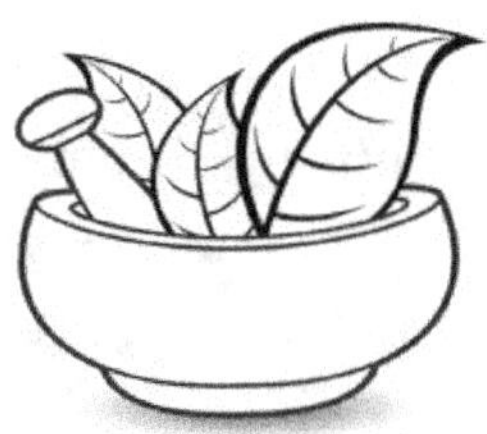

CHAPTER 5

Daily Health Maintenance

As you have decided to take a plunge into this unknown world of herbalism, and truly explore the world of herbal remedies, you would be wise to also try to seamlessly integrate various herbal solutions into your everyday habits. By doing so, you can greatly enhance your health in a vast variety of ways. This chapter is meant to provide you with hands-on methods for bringing these natural aids into your routines, while also highlighting how they can help you stay healthy and ward off sickness. You will discover that with just a bit of intention, you can tap into the wholesome support that herbs provide, thus paving the way for a healthier and more harmonious way of living.

Herbs for Boosting Immunity

For ages, people have turned to herbs as trusted allies in traditional healing, thanks to their remarkable knack for boosting our immune systems and promoting good health. By weaving specific herbs into your everyday life, you are not just strengthening your body's defenses against sickness; you are also nurturing your overall vitality. Let us dive into the unique advantages and applications of three remarkable herbs that we have not previously discussed, namely elderberry, garlic, and Andrographis.

Elderberry

Elderberry is a potent herb known for its immune-enhancing capabilities for it is packed with antioxidants and vitamins A, B, and C, therefore, elderberry supports the immune system and can help shorten the duration of the flu. Research suggests that elderberry may help reduce symptoms of colds and flu and promote quicker recovery (*Dietary Supplements,* 2023). Typically consumed as syrup, capsules, or tea, elderberry's sweet taste also makes it a pleasant addition to your diet. It's important to ensure elderberry products are made from ripe, cooked berries, as the raw fruit can be toxic and cause gastrointestinal distress. Properly manufactured supplements are safe and effective for boosting immunity.

Garlic

Garlic has been used for its medicinal properties for centuries, particularly for its ability to fight bacteria, viruses, and fungi. The key compound in garlic, allicin, is responsible for these antimicrobial effects. Garlic enhances the disease-fighting capabilities of white blood cells and helps the body fend off various infections. While only a few studies have directly examined the effectiveness of garlic against colds and flu, it has been shown to support overall immune function (*Dietary Supplements,* 2023). Fresh garlic can be easily incorporated into your meals, or you can opt for garlic supplements if the strong taste is not appealing. While garlic is generally safe, potential side effects include bad breath and digestive issues. Additionally, those on blood thinners or blood pressure medications should consult a healthcare provider before increasing their garlic intake.

Andrographis

Andrographis, an herb native to Southeast Asia, is renowned for its effectiveness against common colds and flu. It is known to reduce inflammation and is quickly absorbed in tincture form. Studies indicate that Andrographis can lessen the severity of respiratory infection symptoms and may shorten the length of illness (*Dietary Supplements,* 2023). This herb works by stimulating the immune response and has anti-inflammatory properties that can alleviate symptoms like sore throats and fever. Often consumed as a tincture or capsule, Andrographis is a valuable addition to any natural medicine cabinet. However, users should be aware of potential side effects including nausea, dizziness, and fatigue, and it may also interact with blood-thinning medications.

Incorporation

Incorporating these herbs into your daily regimen can be a simple yet effective way to support your immune system. As you explore herbal remedies, you will want to keep in mind the importance of sourcing high-quality products to ensure safety and efficacy. Consulting with a healthcare professional before beginning any new supplement, especially if you have underlying health conditions or are taking other medications, is always advisable.

For elderberry, homemade elderberry syrup is a popular option. You can make it by simmering dried elderberries with water and sweetening it with honey. This syrup can be taken straight by the spoonful or mixed into drinks for a delicious way to fortify your immune system, especially during flu season.

Adding fresh garlic to your dishes is one of the easiest ways to harness its immune-boosting properties. Crush or chop garlic cloves to release the allicin before adding it to sauces, soups, or roasted vegetables. For those who prefer, garlic supplements are available in pill form, providing the benefits without the strong aroma.

Andrographis can be taken as a tincture, which allows for rapid absorption and effectiveness. Adding a few drops to a glass of water or juice can provide a potent dose of this herb when you feel a cold coming on. Capsules offer a more convenient option for daily use, ensuring you receive a consistent amount of the active compounds.

By integrating these immune-supporting herbs into your lifestyle, you are embracing a natural approach to maintaining health and wellness. These remedies serve as complementary practices alongside a balanced diet, regular exercise, and good hygiene habits. Together, they form a holistic strategy for keeping your immune system robust and resilient.

Herbs for Stress Relief and Relaxation

We briefly discussed the benefits of using Ashwagandha to combat stress and promote relaxation in chapter three, but this subject is rather extensive and deserves a deeper examination. Considering that our lives, being part of contemporary society, generate an immense amount of stress for most of us, the various solutions for that should take center stage when discussing our daily health maintenance. Therefore, this section will look at herbs, other than ashwagandha, known for their calming properties, such as lavender, lemon balm, and passionflower.

Calming Lavender

Lavender is one of the most popular herbs used for its calming properties, perhaps because its smell is very pleasant in itself as the essential oil extracted from lavender flowers has a pleasant and soothing aroma that promotes a sense of calmness. Many people use lavender essential oil in aromatherapy to reduce stress and anxiety. Its calming effect also improves sleep quality, making it an excellent remedy for those who suffer from insomnia or restless nights. Additionally, lavender is effective in reducing tension-related headaches.

Lavender, with its calming scent, can be incorporated into daily life through simple yet effective methods such as diffusing essential oils during work hours or adding a few drops to a nighttime bath for ultimate relaxation. Simply inhaling the scent or applying diluted lavender oil to the temples can also provide significant relief. If you wish, creating a tranquil environment with lavender can help you manage anxiety throughout the day and also improve nighttime rest (Curtis, 2024).

Anxiety-Reducing Lemon Balm

Lemon balm, which is another member of the mint family, is celebrated for its ability to reduce anxiety and promote better sleep. Its mild sedative properties make it an ideal choice for those looking to ease the mind and prepare for restful sleep. Lemon balm is also cherished for its light, pleasant flavor, making it suitable for herbal blends and teas. Drinking lemon balm tea before bedtime can create a relaxing nighttime ritual, helping to wind down after a long day. The gentle nature of lemon balm means it can be enjoyed by individuals of all ages, providing a safe option for households looking to incorporate natural calmatives into their routines (*11 Herbs That Can Improve Your Sleep,* 2024).

The versatility of lemon balm makes it particularly appealing. Besides its use in teas, lemon balm can also be incorporated into salads and desserts, offering a delightful way to enjoy its calming benefits. The herb's subtle flavor pairs well with a variety of culinary delights, making it easy to include in numerous meals without overpowering them. Regular consumption of lemon balm can provide consistent support for maintaining a peaceful mind and quality sleep.

Sedative Passionflower

Passionflower is yet another herb renowned for its sedative properties, beneficial for individuals experiencing insomnia or heightened nervousness. Historically, passionflower has been used to treat anxiety and sleep disorders due to its ability to increase gamma-aminobutyric acid (GABA) levels in the brain. GABA slows down brain activity, allowing for a calming effect that facilitates relaxation and sleep. Passionflower can be easily integrated into daily routines; it is available in various forms, including teas, tinctures, and capsules. Including passionflower in your nightly regimen can ensure a smoother transition into sleep, thereby enhancing overall sleep quality (*11 Herbs That Can Improve Your Sleep,* 2024).

The passionflower's effectiveness in easing nervousness and promoting restful sleep cannot be overstated. Including passionflower in your wellness regimen may involve sipping a comforting cup of passionflower tea in the evening or taking a tincture under the tongue before bed. These practices can foster a more restful sleep cycle, ensuring that you wake up refreshed and ready to face the challenges of the day ahead.

Using these herbs daily can aid you as you navigate the stressful waters of life, for it can feel rather impossible to rid yourself of stressors altogether. You should therefore make the effort to incorporate herbs that will aid you through the stress to your daily routine instead.

Enhancing Sleep With Herbal Remedies

Herbs have long been revered for their roles in promoting health and wellness, particularly in the realm of sleep. By incorporating specific herbs into our daily routines, we can improve sleep quality and address common issues related to sleep disturbances. This section will explore how valerian root, hops, magnolia bark, and chamomile can be used effectively to enhance sleep.

Valerian Root

Valerian root stands out as a favored herbal solution for those seeking better sleep, renowned for its ability to shorten the time it takes to fall asleep and enhance sleep quality, all without negative side effects. Sourced from the Valeriana officinalis plant, this natural remedy has been a trusted sedative for centuries. Research suggests that Valerian Root elevates levels of gamma-aminobutyric acid (GABA) in the brain, effectively soothing the nervous system and fostering a sense of calm (*11 Herbs That Can Improve Your Sleep,* 2024). For individuals who find it difficult to drift off or stay asleep, adding Valerian Root to their nightly routine can offer significant advantages. It comes in a variety of forms, including tablets, liquid extracts, and herbal teas, allowing users to choose the method that works best for them.

Hops

Hops, often celebrated for their pivotal role in brewing, possess remarkable calming properties that can significantly enhance sleep quality. In ancient practices, hops were incorporated into pillows, serving as a natural remedy for achieving peaceful slumber. Their chemical constituents function as gentle sedatives, alleviating anxiety and fostering a state of relaxation. The soothing effects of hops make them a superb option for those grappling with stress or sleep disturbances tied to anxiety. When paired with complementary calming herbs like Valerian Root, the advantages of hops can be notably elevated. Drinking hops as a tea or taking it as a supplement before bedtime can cultivate a serene atmosphere, facilitating a smoother journey into restful sleep (*11 Herbs That Can Improve Your Sleep,* 2024).

Magnolia Bark

Magnolia bark serves as a powerful ally for those grappling with sleep issues, especially when these disruptions stem from stress and anxiety. This herb plays a crucial role in regulating cortisol, the stress hormone, fostering a sense of tranquility while alleviating feelings of anxiety (Breus, 2018; Loscalzo, 2023; Weil, 2011). The soothing properties of Magnolia Bark make it invaluable for anyone struggling to relax after a challenging day. Beyond its calming effects, this herb also aids digestion and boasts anti-inflammatory properties, enhancing overall health (Bhattacharya, 2024; Snyder, 2020). By incorporating Magnolia Bark into your nighttime routine—whether as a supplement or a comforting tea—you can pave the way for more profound, restorative sleep.

The Return of Chamomile

Finally, Chamomile, as we have already mentioned several times, is widely celebrated for its gentle yet effective sleep-enhancing properties. It is a versatile herb whose qualities cannot be emphasized enough in terms of effectiveness, and drinking Chamomile tea before bed is a time-honored ritual that not only improves the quality of your sleep but also relaxes your muscles and soothes your mind. Chamomile contains apigenin, an antioxidant that binds to specific receptors in the brain, inducing a sense of calm and reducing insomnia symptoms (*The health benefits of 3 herbal teas,* 2021). Its mild nature makes Chamomile safe for all ages, including children and elderly individuals, offering a holistic approach to better sleep. Whether brewed as a tea or taken in supplement form, Chamomile serves as an accessible and reliable herb for enhancing sleep.

Herbal Antibiotics

Herbal antibiotics are becoming increasingly sought after as more individuals turn to natural remedies to combat bacterial infections, moving away from traditional pharmaceutical options. Such plant-derived solutions, known for their strong antibacterial effects, present an intriguing alternative to standard antibiotics. Therefore, this section will explore what herbal antibiotics entail, their mechanisms of action, and the specific plants recognized for their antibiotic qualities.

Herbal antibiotics stand apart from their conventional counterparts in some important ways. While traditional antibiotics are created in labs to zero in on specific bacteria, herbal options come from whole plants or their extracts and have been used in natural healing for ages. Conventional antibiotics work quickly, often needed for urgent bacterial infections, whereas herbal remedies are generally gentler and may have a more varied effect on the body. This gentleness can result in fewer side effects and less interference with the good bacteria in our gut (Wachtel-Galor & Benzie, 2011).

One of the most well-known herbal antibiotics is garlic. Garlic has been celebrated for its medicinal properties for thousands of years. Modern research validates its efficacy, revealing that compounds such as allicin contribute to its antibacterial effects. Garlic is effective against a range of bacteria, including Salmonella, Escherichia coli (E. coli), and Staphylococcus aureus (S. aureus) (Pietrangelo, 2024). Its broad-spectrum action makes it a valuable tool in fighting bacterial infections. Garlic can be consumed in various forms, including raw, cooked, or as a supplement. However, caution is advised when taking garlic supplements because they have been shown to increase the risk of bleeding. This effect is due to garlic's antiplatelet properties, which can slow down blood clotting. This risk is particularly significant for individuals taking anticoagulant medications or those scheduled for surgery (Cervoni, 2024; *Garlic*, 2020).

Echinacea

This flowering plant, native to North America, has been traditionally used to treat various infections, including respiratory infections and wounds. Its effectiveness lies in its ability to boost the immune system by increasing the activity of white blood cells, which helps the body naturally fend off infections. Research suggests echinacea may lower the risk of respiratory infections, although findings are not entirely consistent across studies (Petre, 2020). Echinacea is available in various forms, including extracts, tinctures, tablets, and capsules. It is typically recommended to use echinacea for no more than ten days to avoid overstimulating the immune system.

Goldenseal

Goldenseal is another herb frequently highlighted for its antibacterial properties. The active compound in goldenseal, berberine, has demonstrated significant antibacterial activities. Berberine works by preventing bacteria from adhering to the walls of the bladder, making it a particularly useful substitute for antibiotics in treating urinary tract infections (UTIs) (Petre, 2020). Despite its effectiveness in laboratory settings, the actual absorption of berberine from goldenseal supplements might be lower compared to concentrated berberine extracts. Therefore, while promising, further research is needed to determine the optimal usage of goldenseal in humans. Goldenseal is commonly combined with echinacea in over-the-counter remedies, yet there's no concrete evidence that this combination provides additional benefits beyond those seen with each herb individually (Petre, 2020).

Thyme and Oregano

Thyme and oregano are also noteworthy for their antibacterial properties. Thyme contains thymol, a compound known for its effectiveness against bacteria such as E. coli and methicillin-resistant S. aureus (MRSA). Oregano oil, rich in carvacrol, has shown promise in combating Streptococcus mutans, a bacterium associated with dental cavities (Pietrangelo, 2024). Both herbs can be used fresh, dried, or in essential oil form, although dosage guidelines for antibiotic use are still under investigation. Incorporating these herbs into your diet can provide a gentle, ongoing defense against harmful bacteria.

How It Works

Understanding the mechanisms through which these herbs combat bacterial infections is crucial. Herbal antibiotics can work in several ways. Some, like garlic, directly attack bacterial cell walls, causing the bacteria to die. Others, like echinacea, enhance the body's immune response, helping the body fight off infections more effectively. Goldenseal's berberine prevents bacteria from sticking to the walls of organs, thereby inhibiting their growth and ability to cause infections. Each herb's unique mechanism contributes to its efficacy and suitability for different types of infections.

However, it is also essential to recognize the benefits and limitations of using herbal antibiotics compared to pharmaceutical ones. One major benefit is the reduced likelihood of developing antibiotic resistance. Pharmaceutical antibiotics, when overused or misused, can lead to bacteria evolving and becoming resistant, rendering these drugs ineffective. Herbal antibiotics, with their broad-spectrum and mild action, are less likely to cause such resistance. Additionally, herbal antibiotics often come with fewer side effects and are generally safer for long-term use.

On the downside, herbal antibiotics may not act as quickly or be as potent as their pharmaceutical counterparts. For severe infections, relying solely on herbal remedies might not provide the necessary level of intervention. It is also critical to use herbal antibiotics correctly and under the guidance of a healthcare provider, especially since some herbs can interact with medications or cause adverse effects in certain individuals.

This chapter has highlighted the remarkable benefits and practical applications of elderberry, garlic, and Andrographis, among a few others, with the sole purpose of aiding you as you learn how to incorporate various herbal remedies into your daily health regimen. As you are now building a foundation of understanding of the unique properties and potential side effects of each herb, you are at this point rather equipped to make informed choices about incorporating them into your health strategies.

It is now time to move on, thus diving into the next chapter that will guide you on how herbs can be used to address specific health concerns. For only by understanding the targeted applications of various herbs, can you deepen your knowledge and refine your approach to holistic health care.

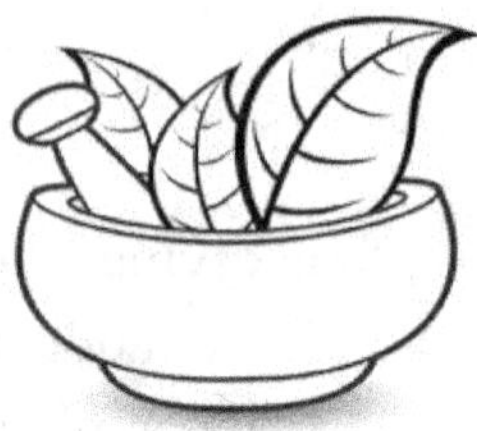

CHAPTER 6

Targeted Treatments

Addressing health concerns with herbal remedies provides a natural pathway to wellness for individuals by focusing on specific issues like pain relief, respiratory support, skin ailments, and women's health. These herbal treatments enable a customized approach to care. This method not only complements holistic health practices but also offers a safer alternative to conventional medications that may come with unwelcome side effects.

Managing Pain and Inflammation

Herbal treatments have been a key part of wellness practices for generations, offering natural approaches to a variety of health issues. Among the diverse array of botanicals, certain herbs are particularly renowned for their pain-relieving and inflammation-reducing effects, proving to be effective options for tackling common discomforts. This section provides insights into the beneficial applications of turmeric, willow bark, ginger, and devil's claw for mitigating pain and decreasing swelling.

Turmeric

This herb has previously been mentioned due to its powerful anti-inflammatory and antioxidant characteristics and has therefore—when incorporated into the diet—been shown to notably improve conditions related to inflammation, such as arthritis and other musculoskeletal disorders. Even having been mentioned before, it is worth mentioning again as scientific studies affirm that curcumin's anti-inflammatory properties are comparable to some pharmaceutical agents, without the adverse side effects common to synthetic medications (Ghasemian et al., 2016).

Understanding the safe use of turmeric is important. It should be noted that curcumin is fat-soluble, meaning it is best absorbed when consumed with fats. Adding a bit of oil or consuming turmeric with meals that contain healthy fats can enhance its bioavailability. One of the easiest ways to include turmeric is through cooking. Dishes like curries, soups, and even smoothies can be enriched with this spice, yielding not only flavor but also health benefits. Additionally, combining turmeric with black pepper increases curcumin absorption due to piperine, a compound found in black pepper that enhances nutrient uptake (Ghasemian et al., 2016).

Willow Bark

Willow bark, revered as "nature's aspirin," contains salicin, a chemical similar to aspirin, making it an effective pain reliever. Historically, it has been utilized for treating headaches, muscle pain, and inflammatory conditions such as bursitis and tendinitis. Modern research supports its efficacy in managing chronic low-back pain and osteoarthritis, though it underscores the importance of understanding its safe use. The typical dosage ranges from 120 to 240 mg of salicin daily, administered for up to eight weeks (*Nutritional Approaches for Musculoskeletal Pain,* 2022).

Willow bark is largely considered safe, but it can lead to some side effects, particularly affecting the digestive system, and it may trigger allergic reactions in a minority of users. Those with a sensitivity to salicylates, individuals with specific medical issues, pregnant women, and children should steer clear of willow bark, as it can pass through the placenta and linger longer in the bodies of newborns. Before embarking on the use of willow bark supplements, it's imperative to consult with healthcare professionals, especially for individuals who are on blood-thinning medications, as this can heighten the risk of bleeding (Shenefelt, 2011).

Ginger

Ginger, celebrated for its warming qualities, is another potent herb for reducing inflammation and pain, but by now you are already aware of the potency of this delicious herb. With its active components gingerol, it has anti-inflammatory and antioxidant effects that are particularly beneficial for joint pain associated with arthritis. Consuming ginger in various forms—fresh, dried, or as a supplement—can help manage symptoms effectively. Fresh ginger can be added to teas, stir-fries, and smoothies, while powdered ginger is a versatile ingredient for baking and seasoning.

Multiple studies have indicated ginger's effectiveness in alleviating pain and improving joint function in individuals with osteoarthritis. For instance, one study demonstrated that taking ginger extract over three months significantly reduced knee pain in participants with osteoarthritis (Ghasemian et al., 2016). Moreover, ginger's ability to inhibit inflammatory pathways without the side effects seen with conventional nonsteroidal anti-inflammatory drugs makes it a valuable addition to a holistic pain management regimen.

Devil's Claw

Devil's claw, a remarkable plant native to Southern Africa, is widely recognized for its ability to alleviate back and joint discomfort. Studies demonstrate its potency in easing arthritis-related pain, thanks to harpagoside—a compound known for its strong anti-inflammatory properties. Available in various forms such as capsules, tablets, and tinctures, devil's claw caters to individual preferences, making it a versatile choice. Ongoing research confirms that regular consumption of this herbal remedy can lead to significant pain relief and enhanced mobility for those grappling with arthritis and lower back issues (Brien et al., 2006).

The safety profile of devil's claw is largely encouraging, but it's crucial to stick to the suggested dosages to steer clear of possible side effects like digestive discomfort. While many people tolerate devil's claw well, individuals with specific health conditions, particularly those involving stomach ulcers or gallstones, should proceed with caution. It's wise to consult a healthcare provider to confirm that it aligns with your current medications and health issues (Brien et al., 2006).

Incorporation

For those new to herbal remedies, starting with culinary applications might be the most accessible entry point. Turmeric, easily added to recipes, provides both flavor and health benefits. Ginger, whether in tea or food, offers a soothing experience along with its therapeutic properties. As familiarity with these herbs grows, exploring supplements and more concentrated forms can further enhance their benefits.

Understanding and respecting the potency of these natural remedies is, however, paramount. While they offer robust benefits, their interactions with other medications and health conditions must be considered. Working with healthcare providers ensures safe and effective integration into one's health regimen.

Herbal Support for Respiratory Health

Targeted treatments with herbal remedies offer a wealth of benefits for individuals seeking natural alternatives to pharmaceuticals, especially in managing specific health concerns. Among these, respiratory support stands out as a critical area where herbs can make a significant impact. We have previously, in chapter three, mentioned thyme, peppermint, and eucalyptus as herbs that aid and support your respiratory health. However, in this chapter, we will mainly gloss over and provide you with a quick recap of those herbs already mentioned but focus mainly on one that has not yet been discussed: lobelia.

Thyme

Thyme is a powerful ally in combating respiratory infections due to its natural antimicrobial properties. For centuries, people have turned to thyme for relief from bronchitis and persistent coughs. Rich in beneficial compounds like thymol, thyme offers antiseptic and antifungal benefits that can ease respiratory issues. Research indicates that thyme can notably reduce cough severity during illness. However, it's crucial to use thyme properly to steer clear of potential risks. Avoid inhaling thyme oil directly, as it's toxic and can lead to severe health complications. Instead, brewing thyme tea or using it in steam inhalation can deliver its benefits safely and effectively (Indigo Herbs, 2014).

Peppermint

Peppermint is a powerful ally for your respiratory health, providing a refreshing sensation that facilitates easier breathing and alleviates sinus pressure. The key component, menthol, helps clear mucus and acts as a soothing expectorant for the throat. It's commonly found in cold medications and throat lozenges due to its effectiveness. Inhaling steam infused with peppermint oil is a practical way to relieve nasal and chest congestion. Yet, be cautious—peppermint oil is not safe for infants and should never be applied directly to their skin, as it can provoke serious reactions (Curtis, 2024).

Eucalyptus

Eucalyptus is renowned for its effective decongestant qualities, often found in chest rubs and steam baths. Its oil appears in numerous cough syrups and lozenges across the U.S. and Europe. By applying eucalyptus ointments to the nose and chest, you can alleviate congestion and break down phlegm. The eucalyptus compounds, like eucalyptol, clear airways and mucus and support lung health naturally. However, caution is advised when using eucalyptus oil around kids, as it can be toxic if ingested. For safe use, steam inhalation is an excellent way to enjoy its benefits (Ruggeri, 2018).

Lobelia

Lobelia is a plant that people use for various health reasons. While it has many benefits, it is important to remember that it can be powerful. Because of this strength, using lobelia often calls for more care compared to other herbs. When we think about using herbs for health, it is easy to overlook how some might be more intense than others. This is where understanding lobelia's unique characteristics becomes essential (Chevallier, 2016).

Lobelia stands out as a lesser known but highly effective herb for respiratory support, particularly in relieving asthma and bronchial spasms. Traditionally used by Native Americans for various medicinal purposes, lobelia is known for its potent alkaloid called lobeline, which has been shown to relax bronchial muscles and thin mucus, making it easier to expel. This makes it beneficial for those suffering from chronic respiratory conditions such as asthma. However, due to its potency, accurate dosing of lobelia is vital. Overdosing can lead to serious side effects such as nausea, vomiting, and even more severe symptoms. Consulting a healthcare provider knowledgeable in herbal medicine is recommended before incorporating lobelia into a treatment regimen (Chevallier, 2016).

The Benefits of Lobelia

Lobelia has been used traditionally for its effects on the respiratory system. For instance, many herbalists recommend it for issues like asthma or bronchitis. It has components that can help with breathing, making it easier for people dealing with these conditions. However, it is important to note that not everyone reacts the same way to lobelia. Some might find it helpful, while others could experience unwanted side effects. This difference in reaction highlights why careful management is necessary when dealing with lobelia (Chevallier, 2016).

Form and Preparation

Lobelia can be used in different forms, such as tinctures, teas, or capsules. Each method of preparation has its own benefits. For instance, tinctures are concentrated liquid extracts and may offer quick relief for respiratory issues. In contrast, teas can be more soothing and easier on the stomach. When deciding how to use lobelia, it is helpful to ask a herbalist about the best form for your specific needs. They can recommend a method that aligns with your lifestyle and preferences (Chevallier, 2016).

The holistic approach offered by these herbal treatments aligns with the growing trend towards sustainable and natural healthcare options. As more individuals seek to minimize their reliance on pharmaceutical drugs due to potential side effects or personal preferences, the accessibility and effectiveness of herbs like thyme, peppermint, eucalyptus, and lobelia become increasingly important. Not only do these plants provide targeted relief, but they also contribute to a broader sense of health autonomy and self-care (Chevallier, 2016).

Natural Remedies for Skin Conditions

When addressing common skin issues like eczema, acne, and minor wounds, certain herbs shine for their remarkable effectiveness and natural advantages. In this section, we will explore how herbal remedies, including aloe vera, calendula, tea tree oil, and lavender, offer holistic solutions, enriching our skincare routines and promoting overall wellness.

Aloe Vera

Aloe Vera is often celebrated as nature's healing ally, cherished for its remarkable soothing properties. This resilient succulent has a long history of effectively addressing various skin concerns, particularly burns and irritations. The magic lies in the gel harvested from its fleshy leaves, abundant in vitamins, minerals, and enzymes that foster skin recovery. When applied to burns, the cooling sensation of aloe vera brings instant comfort and accelerates healing. It also acts as a potent remedy for sunburn, providing a natural solution devoid of harsh chemicals. To fully harness its potential, it's essential to employ proper extraction and application methods. Cutting fresh leaves yields the most genuine aloe gel. Simply slice the leaf open and scoop out the clear gel. Gently apply it to the affected area, allowing your skin to absorb its nourishing properties. Consistent use can dramatically alleviate irritation and minimize burn scars, making aloe vera a vital ingredient in any natural skincare regimen (Brown-Samuels et al., 2024; Shenefelt, 2011).

Calendula

Calendula, often referred to as marigold, stands out as a remarkable ingredient in herbal skincare. Its stunning orange-yellow blooms not only brighten up our surroundings but also offer a wealth of healing properties. Calendula is especially effective in therapeutic ointments and salves designed to mend cuts, scrapes, and minor injuries. With its powerful anti-inflammatory and antiseptic qualities, it promotes faster healing, making it ideal for delicate skin, including that of young children. Additionally, the gentle essence of calendula ensures it won't irritate the skin, solidifying its place in countless natural first-aid kits. To create a calendula ointment, simply infuse dried petals in a carrier oil like olive or coconut oil to draw out their healing goodness. This infused oil can then be blended with beeswax for a calming balm that works wonders on skin abrasions (Brown-Samuels et al., 2024).

Tea Tree Oil

Tea Tree Oil, extracted from the leaves of the Melaleuca alternifolia tree, is well-known for its remarkable antiseptic properties, making it a popular choice for treating acne and fungal infections. Its key component, terpinen-4-ol, effectively combats bacteria and fungi. However, because it's powerful, it's important to use tea tree oil carefully. Diluting it is essential to avoid skin irritation; a widely recommended ratio is 1 part tea tree oil to 20 parts carrier oil, resulting in a safe 5% concentration for topical application. Research has shown that tea tree oil is effective against acne, often leading to fewer side effects like dryness and itching compared to benzoyl peroxide. Additionally, it clears blemishes gently without the harshness of synthetic chemicals. Applying diluted tea tree oil directly to problem areas can help reduce inflammation and eradicate acne-causing bacteria, resulting in clearer skin over time. Its antifungal characteristics also make it an excellent choice for conditions such as athlete's foot and nail fungus (Brown-Samuels et al., 2024).

Lavender in Short

As we have already touched base on lavender several times, the only thing worth adding to that, related to this topic, is the fact that lavender oil, distilled from the flowers, contains active compounds like linalool and linalyl acetate, which exhibit anti-inflammatory and antimicrobial effects. These properties make lavender especially effective for treating minor burns, insect bites, and various skin irritations. Adding a few drops of lavender oil to your bathwater can not only help you relax but also soothe irritated skin. Similarly, incorporating lavender-infused lotions or creams into daily skincare can enhance your skin health while also providing stress relief through its aromatic qualities; a win-win situation of sorts.

Using Herbs for Women's Health

Herbs have been employed for centuries to promote women's health, providing natural solutions for various concerns related to menstrual health, menopause symptoms, and reproductive health. This segment focuses on the practical applications of four key herbs: Chaste Tree Berry (Vitex), Red Clover, Evening Primrose Oil, and Nettle. These herbs offer targeted treatments that can address specific issues effectively, fostering holistic well-being among women.

Chaste Tree Berry (Vitex)

Chaste Tree Berry, commonly referred to as Vitex, is highly regarded for its potent effects on menstrual regulation and for easing the discomfort of premenstrual syndrome (PMS). This herb has a rich history in traditional healing practices, primarily influencing the pituitary gland to promote hormonal harmony. For women facing challenges like erratic cycles or severe PMS—marked by emotional fluctuations, abdominal bloating, and tenderness in the breasts—Vitex may offer a welcome source of relief and balance (Kenda et al., 2021).

Dosage is vital for the safe and effective use of Chaste Tree Berry. For most individuals, a daily intake of 20–40 mg of standardized extract is advisable. While it may take a few months of regular use to see noticeable changes, dedication often leads to remarkable advantages. It's wise to consult a healthcare provider before embarking on any herbal regimen, ensuring it aligns with your unique health circumstances and avoids possible interactions with other medications (Kenda et al., 2021).

Red Clover

Red Clover stands out as an exceptional herb that promotes women's health, especially during the transition of menopause. Rich in phytoestrogens, Red Clover includes natural compounds that emulate estrogen in the body, offering a supportive ally for those grappling with menopause symptoms like hot flashes, night sweats, and emotional fluctuations (Kenda et al., 2021).

Scientific research indicates that Red Clover serves as an effective ally for women navigating the aging process, promoting hormonal balance while also enhancing cardiovascular health and bone strength. For optimal benefits, a daily intake of 40–80 mg of isoflavone extract is often recommended. As with any herbal remedy, it's crucial to follow recommended dosages and consult with a healthcare professional to ensure that the treatment aligns with individual health needs and conditions (Kenda et al., 2021).

Evening Primrose Oil

Evening Primrose Oil is renowned for its rich concentration of gamma-linolenic acid (GLA), a vital omega-6 fatty acid known for its anti-inflammatory effects. Many turn to this oil to alleviate the discomforts associated with PMS, such as mood fluctuations, breast tenderness, and bloating. Furthermore, Evening Primrose Oil enhances skin vitality, effectively addressing conditions like eczema and acne, which may flare up due to hormonal shifts (Kenda et al., 2021).

Properly using Evening Primrose Oil is crucial for achieving its full benefits. Most people find that a daily intake of 500–1000 mg works well, but it's wise to start with a smaller amount and gradually increase it to see how your body reacts. Some individuals might notice mild digestive issues at first, but these often lessen as your body adjusts. To really maximize the positive effects of Evening Primrose Oil, consider incorporating it into a balanced diet and making healthy lifestyle choices, as this combination can significantly amplify its advantages (Kenda et al., 2021).

Nettle

Nettle is a powerhouse of nutrients, offering a wide range of benefits for overall women's health. This herb is rich in vitamins A, C, K, and several B vitamins, along with minerals such as iron, calcium, magnesium, and potassium. During pregnancy, Nettle can provide essential nutritional support, promoting both maternal health and fetal development (Chevallier, 2016).

However, caution is advised when using Nettle, especially for those with specific health conditions like kidney disease or allergies to plants in the Urticaceae family. The typical dose involves consuming Nettle leaf tea or taking 300–600 mg of dried leaf extract daily. Due to its potent diuretic properties, ensuring adequate hydration while using Nettle is crucial to prevent dehydration (Chevallier, 2016).

Integrating Herbal Remedies Into Daily Routines

Incorporating these herbs into daily routines can be both simple and rewarding. Herbal teas, tinctures, capsules, and topical applications offer various convenient methods of consumption. Combining these herbs with a balanced diet, regular exercise, and stress management techniques can amplify their effects, contributing to a holistic approach to women's health.

Chaste Tree Berry, with its hormone-regulating properties, can be easily integrated into a morning routine by taking a standardized extract supplement. Red Clover can be enjoyed as a soothing tea, providing both relaxation and symptom relief. Evening Primrose Oil capsules can be taken alongside meals to aid absorption and minimize potential gastrointestinal discomfort. Nettle, available in both tea and supplement forms, can be consumed daily to maintain overall vitality.

Herbs provide a natural and effective way to support women's health throughout different life stages, offering solutions for concerns related to menstrual health, menopause, and reproductive wellness. By understanding and utilizing herbs like Chaste Tree Berry, Red Clover, Evening Primrose Oil, and Nettle, women can address specific health issues with personalized herbal treatments. The importance of proper dosage and administration cannot be overstated, making it crucial to consult healthcare providers to tailor herbal therapies to individual needs.

This chapter has explored the practical applications of key herbal remedies for managing specific health challenges and understanding the safe and effective use of these herbs is vital for optimizing their benefits. You are encouraged to start with simple culinary applications and gradually explore more concentrated forms such as supplements or topical treatments. Consulting healthcare providers before integrating any herbal remedies ensures safe use, particularly for individuals on other medications or with existing health conditions. On this topic, however, we will move on to the next chapter which discusses the precautions necessary when using herbal remedies. This chapter will guide you as you learn how to identify potential risks, aid you in understanding interactions with medications, and thereby make it possible for you to make informed decisions to ensure the safe and effective use of herbs in your, and others', daily life.

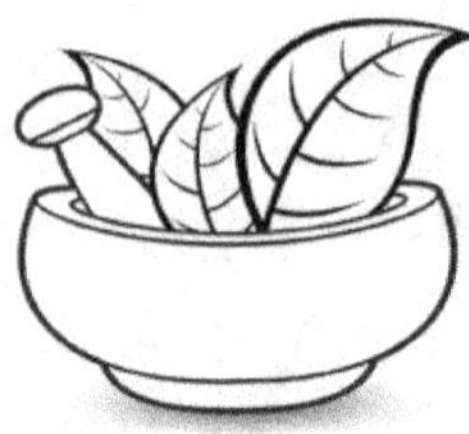

CHAPTER 7

Safety and Contraindications

Ensuring the safe use of herbal remedies is a crucial aspect as you venture down the road of mastering herbal remedies. Understanding the potential risks and adverse effects is essential for anyone considering incorporating herbs into their health regimen, and you must therefore pay close attention while working with your herbs. While many people believe that natural products are inherently safe, it is important to recognize that herbs can cause side effects or interact with other medications. This chapter explores the significance of safety and contraindications associated with herbal remedies where you will learn, among other things, about common allergic reactions to various herbs and how these can range from mild skin irritations to severe conditions like anaphylaxis. This chapter aims to raise awareness and provide you with practical advice for safely integrating herbal remedies into your health routine.

Potential Side Effects and Allergies

Understanding Allergic Reactions to Herbal Remedies

Allergic responses to herbal substances can differ greatly, ranging from mild skin irritations to potentially fatal reactions. Typical allergies linked to herbs often present as skin rashes or contact dermatitis, appearing when the skin interacts with a triggering herb. For instance, those sensitive to ragweed may also experience reactions to chamomile, as both belong to the same botanical family. These allergic responses can vary widely from simple irritations to more intense symptoms such as hives or breathing difficulties.

Anaphylaxis

Anaphylaxis is a life-threatening reaction that, while uncommon, demands immediate recognition. This serious condition presents with alarming symptoms like shortness of breath, facial or throat swelling, and a swift decrease in blood pressure. For instance, those allergic to the daisy family may experience anaphylaxis due to echinacea. Individuals need to understand their allergies and possible reactions to various plants, seeking guidance from healthcare professionals whenever there is uncertainty about the safety of an herb (Ekor, 2014).

Typical Side Effects of Herbal Remedies

Numerous herbal treatments, despite being derived from natural sources, can lead to side effects that mirror those of traditional medications. Digestive issues often arise, such as nausea, vomiting, diarrhea, and stomach discomfort. For instance, large quantities of aloe vera can function as a potent laxative, resulting in significant digestive turmoil. Likewise, excessive consumption of ginseng can irritate the stomach lining, potentially causing nausea or diarrhea.

Skin reactions often emerge as a common adverse effect. When using topical herbs like tea tree oil, some may experience redness, itching, or blisters, especially those with sensitive skin. Although less frequently encountered, dizziness from certain herbs warrants attention; for instance, excessive consumption of kava may result in feelings of vertigo or light-headedness. By recognizing these potential side effects, you can make well-informed choices about integrating herbal remedies into your wellness practices (Ewumi, 2022).

Assessing Risk Factors

Herbal remedies can affect people differently based on their unique health conditions. For instance, those with preexisting liver issues should approach hepatotoxic herbs, like kava and comfrey, with caution, as these may worsen liver problems. Similarly, those with heart conditions must be vigilant about herbs that influence heart health, such as licorice root, which has the potential to increase blood pressure.

Concurrent treatments, including prescribed medications, are crucial for effective health management. Certain herbs can disrupt how these drugs are processed in the body, potentially diminishing their effectiveness or heightening their toxicity. For instance, St. John's Wort is well-known for its capacity to lessen the potency of several medications, such as contraceptives and antidepressants. Consequently, it's essential for those who are on medication to discuss any plans to incorporate herbal supplements with their healthcare providers.

What to Do if You Experience a Reaction

If an adverse reaction occurs, it's essential to assess the severity of symptoms. For mild reactions, like minor rashes or gastrointestinal discomfort, discontinuing the herb and monitoring symptoms might suffice. However, any signs of a severe reaction, such as difficulty breathing, severe dizziness, or swelling, warrant immediate medical attention. In such cases, calling emergency services or going directly to the nearest hospital is crucial.

Reporting adverse effects to healthcare providers ensures accurate medical records and helps identify harmful interactions or allergies. It's also helpful to use resources like *MedWatch*, the FDA's Safety Information and Adverse Event Reporting Program, to document serious problems related to herbal remedies (*Reporting Serious Problems to*

FDA, 2020). This reporting not only aids in personal health management but also contributes to broader public health knowledge by identifying patterns of adverse reactions.

Building Awareness and Seeking Professional Guidance

Raising awareness about the potential dangers linked to herbal remedies is crucial. Many mistakenly believe that natural products are always safe, which isn't necessarily true. Through public education initiatives and easily accessible resources, we can guide users on how to effectively incorporate herbal remedies into their wellness routines. By taking straightforward steps, such as trying one new herb at a time, people can carefully observe any reactions without overwhelming confusion.

Professional advice from experienced herbalists or healthcare practitioners can greatly reduce potential risks. These experts can tailor recommendations based on an individual's unique health background and ongoing treatments. They also serve as trustworthy fountains of knowledge and can guide you toward safe, research-supported herbal methods. Seeking guidance from a professional is especially crucial when navigating complicated health issues or considering herbs that have strong physiological effects.

Interactions With Pharmaceutical Medications

Understanding the interaction between herbal remedies and prescription or over-the-counter medications is crucial for anyone looking to incorporate herbs into their health regimen. Herbal remedies can significantly affect how conventional medications work, sometimes enhancing their effects (potentiation) or diminishing them (antagonism). For instance, St. John's Wort is a popular herb often used for its antidepressant properties, but it can interact with prescription antidepressants, leading to potentially dangerous levels of serotonin in the body. This type of interaction underscores the importance of awareness and caution when combining herbal remedies with other treatments.

Another critical aspect to consider is the specific herbs known to commonly interact with medications. Garlic, for example, has cardiovascular benefits but can interact with blood thinners like warfarin, increasing the risk of bleeding. It's essential to consult healthcare professionals before combining such herbs with medications. They can provide guidance on whether these combinations are safe and, if so, under what conditions they should be taken. Consulting healthcare providers can prevent adverse reactions and ensure the effectiveness of both the herbal remedy and the medication (Asher, Corbett, & Hawke, 2017).

Timing

The timing of taking herbal remedies alongside medications is another key factor. Administering herbs and medicines at the correct times can mitigate potential interactions. For example, taking an herb several hours apart from medication can reduce the risk of interaction by allowing the body to metabolize each substance separately. This practice can be particularly important for those who are on multiple medications or those using herbs that have potent effects on drug absorption and metabolism.

Keeping detailed records of all supplements and medications is also vital. Maintaining a comprehensive list of everything consumed, including dosages and timings, helps manage potential interactions. Sharing this information with healthcare providers ensures they have a complete picture of your regimen, allowing them to offer the best advice and make any necessary adjustments to avoid interactions. Communication with healthcare providers about all aspects of one's health regimen fosters a partnership that prioritizes safety and efficacy (Asher, Corbett, & Hawke, 2017).

Safe Dosages and Administration Guidelines

Incorporating herbal remedies into your wellness routine can yield significant rewards, provided that you pay careful attention to safety precautions, especially when it comes to dosages and methods of use. Knowing how to accurately assess dosages for different herbal solutions is essential to minimize any risks and enhance the advantages they offer.

Understanding Dosage Principles

To start, determining safe dosages for herbal remedies involves several key factors, such as age, weight, and overall health. Children and adults metabolize substances differently, so their dosage requirements vary significantly. For example, what might be appropriate for an adult could be overly intense for a child or an older adult. Additionally, those with certain medical conditions may require customized dosages. Those people suffering from liver or kidney concerns, for instance, often need to take lower doses since their bodies handle medications differently. It's crucial to keep these personal considerations in mind before settling on a dosage.

Another important factor in assessing safe dosages is the type of herbal remedy used. Herbal products are available in many formats, including teas, capsules, tinctures, and extracts, each with its own concentration levels. Grasping these distinctions is crucial for effective dosing. Typically, teas provide a gentler effect compared to capsules or tinctures, which pack a stronger punch. Consequently, a teaspoon of herb in tea form is not equivalent to a teaspoon of its tincture. When combining different forms, it is vital to measure accurately and standardize dosages to guarantee effectiveness while avoiding the risk of overdose (Ewumi, 2022).

Common Dosage Forms

The different forms of herbal remedies necessitate varying dosage considerations. Teas, commonly used for their soothing properties, are typically consumed in larger volumes but contain lower concentrations of active ingredients. On the other hand, capsules and tablets offer precise dosages since they are pre-measured. These forms are convenient for those who need consistent and easily administered doses. Tinctures, made by soaking herbs in alcohol or vinegar, are highly concentrated and thus require careful measurement, often in drops rather than teaspoons or tablespoons.

Measuring and standardizing dosages helps maintain consistency and effectiveness. For instance, using standardized herbal extracts ensures that each dose contains a set number of active compounds, leading to reliable therapeutic effects. This is particularly important for herbs with potent active ingredients where slight variations in dosage can significantly alter their impact.

Signs of Overdose

Recognizing the symptoms of an overdose is critical for anyone using herbal remedies. Symptoms can vary depending on the herb, but common signs include nausea, dizziness, headaches, swelling, upset stomach, and difficulty breathing. More severe symptoms might involve confusion, loss of consciousness, or convulsions, indicating a medical emergency. If you suspect an overdose, it's imperative to act quickly. Contact emergency services immediately, especially if symptoms escalate rapidly (*Drug overdose*, 2012).

There are clear guidelines for responding to an overdose. Firstly, do not induce vomiting unless instructed by a healthcare professional. Instead, try to remain calm and call for medical assistance. Providing activated charcoal, under professional guidance, can help absorb some of the toxins in the digestive tract. However, always follow up with a healthcare provider to ensure complete and safe management of the situation. Learning these first-aid measures can make a crucial difference in preventing serious outcomes from an overdose (*Drug overdose*, 2012).

Consulting Professional Resources

Relying on reputable sources is essential when navigating the intricate landscape of safe and effective dosages. Engaging with literature, analyzing clinical research, and consulting with experienced herbalists or healthcare professionals can provide critical guidance. Titles such as *Medical Herbalism* (Hoffmann, 2003) and *Herbal Medicine: Expanded Commission E Monographs* (Blumenthal, Goldberg & Brinckmann, 2002) serve as valuable compendiums, delivering in-depth information on the applications and dosage recommendations for a variety of herbs, making them indispensable tools for anyone interested in herbal practices.

Consulting a healthcare professional, such as a licensed naturopathic doctor or an experienced herbalist, is also crucial. These professionals can personalize dosage recommendations based on individual health profiles and ongoing treatments. For example, they can adjust dosages for someone taking prescription medication to avoid harmful interactions (Ewumi, 2022). Their expertise helps bridge the gap between traditional knowledge and modern science, ensuring the safe and effective use of herbal medicines.

Online databases and peer-reviewed journals also provide valuable insights into herbal remedies and their proper dosages. Resources like PubMed grant access to a wealth of scientific articles that explore clinical trials and studies focused on herbal medicine. By tapping into these resources, you can remain updated on the latest discoveries and refine their practices accordingly.

Practical Guidelines for Safe Dosage

To ensure the safe use of herbal remedies, here are some practical guidelines:

1. **Start Low and Go Slow**: Begin with the lowest recommended dose and gradually increase until the desired effect is achieved. This approach minimizes the risk of adverse reactions.

2. **Monitor Responses**: Keep track of any changes in health or side effects experienced. Maintaining a journal can help identify patterns and adjust dosages, as necessary.

3. **Avoid Self-Prescribing**: Consult a healthcare professional before starting any new herbal remedy, especially if you have existing health conditions or take other medications.

4. **Follow Instructions Carefully**: Adhere strictly to dosage instructions provided on product labels or by a healthcare provider. Never exceed the recommended dose.

Importance of Professional Guidance

Incorporating herbal remedies into a health regimen requires careful consideration and guidance from healthcare professionals, particularly herbalists. Herbalists are trained experts who specialize in the use of plants for medicinal purposes. They provide invaluable knowledge on the safe and effective use of herbs, considering an individual's unique health profile and needs. The guidance provided by herbalists often adheres to peer-reviewed practices, ensuring that recommendations are based on sound scientific evidence and traditional knowledge. This approach helps minimize risks and maximizes the therapeutic benefits of herbal remedies.

The value of consulting with a professional cannot be overstated. Herbalists can offer personalized advice, identify potential interactions with other medications, and suggest suitable dosages. This individualized attention is crucial because different herbs contain specific chemical compounds that can have varying effects on the body. For instance, echinacea is commonly used to boost the immune system, while ginger aids in digestion, and ginkgo biloba supports cognitive function (Karsch-Völk et al., 2014; Sharifi-Rad et al., 2017). Given these diverse effects, professional guidance ensures that the chosen remedies align with the user's overall health strategy.

An integrative approach to health, which combines conventional and alternative therapies, can offer a more holistic path to wellness. Evidence suggests that collaborative healthcare methods, where herbalists work alongside doctors and other healthcare providers, yield better outcomes. For example, integrative medicine approaches seek to combine the best practices from traditional and modern medicine to provide comprehensive and personalized healthcare solutions (Wang et al., 2023).

Finding reputable herbalists and healthcare providers who respect and understand herbal medicine is essential for safe usage. When searching for such professionals, it is important to ask the right questions to gauge their expertise. Inquire about their qualifications, training, and experience with herbal medicine. Ask if they adhere to peer-reviewed practices and request references or testimonials from previous clients. This diligence helps ensure that the chosen practitioner is knowledgeable and capable of providing reliable advice.

To aid in this process, here are some tips for identifying qualified professionals:

1. **Verify Credentials**: Ensure the herbalist has relevant certifications and licenses from recognized institutions.

2. **Experience Matters**: Look for practitioners with significant experience and a track record of successful patient outcomes.

3. **Ask About Practices**: Understand their approach to integrating herbal remedies with conventional treatments.

4. **Seek Recommendations**: Get referrals from trusted sources, such as healthcare providers or fellow users of herbal medicine.

5. **Consultation**: Schedule an initial consultation to discuss your health goals and see if their philosophy aligns with yours.

Support System

Building a support system that includes healthcare providers, herbalists, and other trusted resources fosters open communication regarding herbal use. This network ensures a cohesive health strategy where all aspects of one's health are considered. Open dialogue between all parties allows for the monitoring of progress and the prompt addressing of any adverse effects.

Establishing a strong support network involves several steps:

1. **Communicate with Your Primary Care Physician**: Keep your doctor informed about your interest in herbal remedies and discuss how they can fit into your current health plan.

2. **Collaborate with Specialists**: If you have a specific condition, consult specialists who may offer insights into how herbal remedies can complement your treatment.

3. **Join Support Groups**: Participate in communities or groups focused on herbal medicine where you can share experiences and recommendations.

4. **Utilize Professional Networks**: Leverage professional networks of healthcare providers who collaborate with herbalists.

By fostering open communication and collaboration, you can achieve a balanced and informed approach to using herbal remedies. Such an approach mitigates risks, leverages the strengths of both traditional and modern medical practices, and promotes optimal health outcomes.

Understanding the potential risks and adverse effects associated with herbal remedies is crucial for anyone looking to incorporate these natural options into their health routine. As this chapter has emphasized the importance of recognizing common allergic reactions and typical side effects, you should feel a bit more certain of the potential signs of severe reactions and know the steps to take if they occur. Now, moving on to the next chapter, we will explore how to source and use herbs responsibly. This includes understanding the environmental impact of herbal harvesting and cultivation and adopting practices that ensure the long-term availability of these valuable resources. By embracing sustainable herbal practices, you can support your health while also contributing to the health of our planet.

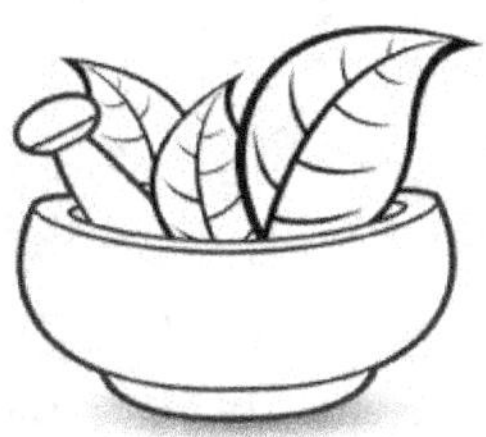

CHAPTER 8

Sustainable Herbal Practices

Sustainable herbal practices encompass a broad range of ethical and environmental considerations essential for anyone involved in herbal remedies. Ethical sourcing ensures that the gathering of herbs does not negatively impact their natural habitats or lead to the depletion of plant species. Being environmentally conscious means utilizing methods that nurture the ecosystem, including responsible harvesting techniques and embracing organic farming approaches. Throughout this chapter, we will explore the various practices that embody sustainable herbalism and emphasize the importance of adhering to Good Agricultural Practices (GAP) to maintain high-quality herb production while safeguarding the environment.

Sustainable Harvesting Techniques

Foraging Laws

For sustainable herb harvesting practices that protect plant populations and preserve ecological harmony, it is crucial to start with a clear grasp of the various foraging regulations. Therefore, you will have to do a bit of research so that you are aware of the local guidelines regarding the collection of wild plants, for only then can you truly honor the limits of nature. Many areas have established specific laws that are aimed at shielding particular plant species from excessive gathering and ensuring the ecosystem remains unharmed. Knowing these rules not only safeguards the natural world but also helps avoid any legal issues for the forager. To become acquainted with these regulations, you can review community statutes or engage with nearby conservation organizations, for these regulations vary a great deal depending on where in the world you reside and we could create an entire book on merely this topic, were we to try and attempt to put all of these regulations together.

Best Practices for Harvesting

Once you feel comfortable with the legal aspects of harvesting in your surroundings, you should dig deep and focus on the best practices for harvesting. Techniques like selective pruning and limiting the amount gathered in a specific area are truly valuable in encouraging plant resilience.

Selective Pruning

Selective pruning involves carefully choosing which parts of the plant to collect, ensuring that the plant can continue to grow and thrive after parts are harvested. For instance, when gathering leaves or flowers, harvesters should avoid taking more than one-third of the plant. This practice helps the plant retain enough foliage or blooms to photosynthesize and reproduce (Chen et al., 2016).

Gathering Limitations

Limiting the amount gathered in a specific area is another critical technique. Over-harvesting from one spot can deplete that area's resources and take a long time to recover. By spreading out the collection points and only taking small amounts from each location, the plants have a better chance to replenish themselves. This method supports the overall ecological balance and prevents the decline of local herb populations (Chen, 2016).

Seasonal Harvesting

Seasonal harvesting insights are very important for enhancing both the efficacy of herbs and their long-term viability. Understanding the ideal times to gather specific herbs ensures a richer yield and promotes sustainable practices. For instance, the leaves of many plants reach their peak potency in spring when the life force of the plant is dedicated to new growth. Similarly, flowers should be picked just shy of their full bloom to harness their highest medicinal value. Roots, however, are best unearthed in the fall, once the visible parts of the plant have died back, as this is when energy has transferred to the subterranean parts (Chen, 2016).

This knowledge of seasonal cycles helps ensure that the harvested herbs are at their peak effectiveness and supports sustainable practices. Collecting herbs at the wrong time not only diminishes their medicinal value but can also stress the plant and its environment.

Innovation

Innovative methods for gathering herbs are transforming the approach to sustainable collection entirely. Utilizing tools that reduce damage to plants while enhancing ecological balance can significantly impact our environment. One effective strategy involves mapping the locations of herb populations to safeguard against over-harvesting. By employing Geographic Information Systems (GIS) and advanced mapping technologies, gatherers can monitor their collection areas and pinpoint regions that require recovery time. This technique helps avert excessive harvesting, allowing ecosystems to rejuvenate and thrive (Katumo et al., 2022).

Another innovative tool is the use of specialized pruners and harvesters that cause minimal damage to the plants. These tools are designed to make clean cuts that do not harm the plant's ability to regenerate. For example, some devices can gently shake seeds loose without damaging the stems or roots, ensuring that the plant can continue to grow after harvesting (Mutterspaugh, 2024).

Good Agricultural Practices (GAP)

Enhancing sustainable harvesting can also be achieved by implementing Good Agricultural Practices (GAP). GAP offers detailed guidelines that oversee production, guarantee quality, and standardize herbal medications. These practices focus on creating premium, safe, and eco-friendly herbal products by utilizing existing knowledge to solve various challenges. GAP addresses key areas such as the environmental conditions of growing sites, plant genetics, farming techniques, harvesting methods, and quality assurance protocols like pesticide testing, chemical analysis of active ingredients, and checks for heavy metals (Chen et al., 2016).

Countries such as China are taking active steps to implement GAP for the cultivation of widely used herbal medicines in areas where these plants have deep-rooted significance. The organic farming approach integrated into GAP focuses on producing high-quality herbal materials while promoting the conservation and sustainable use of these vital plants. A key feature of organic farming is the ban on synthetic fertilizers, pesticides, and herbicides, which corresponds with the stringent organic certification requirements found in Europe and North America. By employing organic fertilizers, farmers can consistently nourish the soil and enhance its stability, leading to healthier growth of medicinal plants and improved production of important bioactive compounds (Chen et al., 2016).

Organic fertilizers significantly boost the biomass output of Chrysanthemum balsamita and improve its essential oil production compared to those cultivated without these nutrients. Such methods play a vital role in nurturing the ongoing growth and sustainability of medicinal plants, fostering compassionate production systems, ecologically sound, and economically viable (Chen et al., 2016).

Supporting Ethical Herb Suppliers

In today's fast-paced world, the demand for herbal products is growing as more people seek natural alternatives for health and wellness.

However, with this surge comes the responsibility to ensure that these products are sourced ethically and sustainably.

Ethical Suppliers

One of the first steps in promoting sustainable herbal practices is identifying ethical suppliers. When evaluating herbal suppliers, considering their transparency in sourcing and production processes is crucial. This transparency is evident when companies provide clear information about where and how they source their herbs. For example, Gaia Herbs emphasizes the importance of sourcing ingredients in conditions and climates that allow herbs to reach their fullest potential (*Ethical Sourcing,* 2022). Look for suppliers who openly share details about their farming practices, partnerships, and testing procedures to ensure product purity and potency.

Fair Trade and Organic Farming

Another important criterion is whether the suppliers adhere to fair trade principles and support organic farming methods or not. Companies that prioritize organic and fair trade practices not only contribute to environmental sustainability but also ensure the well-being of the communities involved in herb cultivation. These suppliers often go beyond organic certifications by implementing biodynamic and regenerative organic practices that emphasize soil health and biodiversity (*Ethical Sourcing,* 2022).

Local Businesses and Directly Engaging With Suppliers

Supporting local suppliers offers numerous benefits worth exploring. By choosing to shop locally, we can significantly decrease the environmental impact caused by extended shipping distances. This practice also ensures that we enjoy fresher products, which is crucial for the effectiveness of herbal solutions. When you buy from nearby sources, you play an active role in bolstering your community's economy and empowering small-scale farmers to succeed. Moreover, local vendors tend to be more transparent about their operations, facilitating a deeper understanding of their dedication to sustainable practices.

Engaging directly with suppliers is another effective way to ensure long-term sustainability in herbal sourcing. Open communication allows consumers to ask critical questions about the origins of ingredients and the methods used in harvesting and processing. When engaging with suppliers, inquire about their environmental impact, labor practices, and commitment to regenerative agriculture. For instance, Ethic Herbs provides detailed ingredient sourcing information on their website and encourages open dialogue with customers, fostering transparency and trust (Galan, 2024). Such interactions not only build trust but also push suppliers to maintain high ethical standards in their operations.

Advocating for Change

Advocating for change within the herbal industry is a compelling way to contribute to broader movements that seek to better ethical practices. By raising awareness and holding companies accountable, you as the consumer can play a significant role in shaping industry standards. Getting involved in campaigns and backing organizations focused on sustainable farming and fair trade helps amplify your message. For example, supporting certifications like USDA Organic or Fair Trade ensures that suppliers follow strict environmental and social guidelines. Your efforts can inspire more companies to embrace eco-friendly practices, ultimately fostering a positive transformation within the industry.

Creating a more sustainable herbal market requires collective effort. By aligning your purchasing decisions with ethical standards, you are not only protecting your health but also contributing to preserving the resources of our planet. Identifying ethical suppliers involves scrutinizing their transparency and commitment to fair trade and organic practices. Supporting local suppliers reduces environmental impact and fosters community growth. Engaging with suppliers through direct communication ensures that ethical practices are maintained. Finally, advocating for change empowers consumers to drive the industry towards more sustainable and responsible methods.

Growing Your Own Herbs Organically

Growing your herbs through organic methods not only lessens dependence on commercial vendors but also offers a wealth of advantages for both you and the ecosystem. A key benefit of cultivating herbs at home is the ability to dictate the growing environment, leading to robust plants devoid of harmful substances. By steering clear of artificial pesticides and fertilizers, you enhance the surrounding ecosystem and yield superior herbs that are both safe and nourishing.

Organic

Organic gardening practices are vital for nurturing a thriving herb garden. At the core of successful organic cultivation lies the management of soil health. Soil brimming with organic matter fosters a rich ecosystem of microorganisms that contribute to vigorous plant development. You can boost soil vitality by incorporating compost, which transforms kitchen scraps and yard waste into nutrient-dense humus. Composting not only revitalizes the soil but also helps minimize waste in landfills.

Pest Control

Another important element of organic gardening is the use of natural methods for pest management. Rather than depending on synthetic pesticides, why not attract helpful insects like ladybugs, which feast on aphids and similar nuisances? Additionally, employing companion planting—where specific plants are cultivated in proximity to mutually benefit each other—can significantly reduce the presence of unwanted pests. For instance, growing marigolds alongside your herbs can effectively fend off nematodes and whiteflies.

Water Conservation

Water conservation is another vital practice in organic gardening. Efficient watering methods like drip irrigation ensure water is delivered directly to plant roots, minimizing evaporation and runoff. Mulching with organic materials such as straw or wood chips helps retain soil moisture, suppress weeds, and eventually decompose to enrich the soil.

Limited Space

For those facing spatial constraints, cultivating herbs in pots or elevated garden beds presents a viable alternative. Container gardening enables you to nurture your herbs on terraces, balconies, or even your kitchen window. This approach offers the convenience of shifting plants to ideal spots according to light and weather patterns. Elevated beds serve as another superb choice, particularly for those dealing with subpar soil or physical challenges. They provide improved drainage and can be filled with nutrient-rich soil specifically designed to meet the unique requirements of your herbs.

Community gardens present yet another alternative for those who lack private gardening space. These shared spaces not only provide an opportunity to grow herbs but also foster community spirit and shared knowledge among gardeners. Participating in a community garden allows you to benefit from collective resources and expertise while contributing to a larger environmental effort.

Attention and Care

Cultivating a thriving herb garden takes continual effort and dedication. One essential technique is crop rotation, which involves switching out the varieties of plants you cultivate in a given spot each season. This method not only prevents the exhaustion of nutrients in the soil but also minimizes the risk of pests and diseases that are specific to certain plants. By varying the crops, you promote a variety of root systems that enhance soil aeration and allow for better absorption of nutrients.

Companion planting complements the practice of crop rotation. Some plants thrive when paired together, promoting each other's growth and warding off pests. For example, when you cultivate basil alongside tomatoes, it can deter harmful pests like aphids, mosquitoes, and the notorious tomato hornworm. Likewise, chamomile enhances the essential oil production of nearby herbs, increasing their medicinal potency.

Seasonal care is essential for maintaining a flourishing herb garden throughout the year. As spring arrives, concentrate on enriching your garden beds with compost and loosening the soil. This is also the perfect opportunity to start seeds indoors or buy young plants for transferring to their new home in the garden. Summer represents the height of growth, making regular watering, weeding, and pest management vital to your garden's success. With the arrival of fall, embrace the cooler temperatures by planting resilient herbs that will thrive through winter, and don't forget to add a layer of mulch to shield the soil and roots from the chill.

Winter is not a season to abandon gardening; rather, it presents a chance to strategize for the upcoming growing period. Within the comfort of your home, you can cultivate herbs on sunlit windowsills or beneath grow lights. Indoor gardening not only lets you savor fresh herbs throughout the year but also allows you to experiment with different varieties and techniques in a dynamic environment.

The journey to sustainable herb gardening begins with small steps— starting a compost pile, setting up a rain barrel, or simply planting a few herbs in containers. Over time, these efforts accumulate, leading to a lush, sustainable herb garden that provides fresh, healthy herbs for your culinary and medicinal needs.

Contributing to Biodiversity Preservation

Understanding Biodiversity

Biodiversity is the variety of life in the world or a particular habitat or ecosystem. In herbal practices, maintaining biodiversity is crucial for ecosystem balance and health. Diverse plant populations contribute to a resilient ecosystem that can withstand environmental changes and disruptions. For instance, different plants support various animal species, including insects, birds, and mammals. Each species plays a unique role, such as pollination, seed dispersal, or soil aeration, which maintains the ecological equilibrium.

In natural ecosystems, biodiversity ensures the stability of food webs and nutrient cycles. A diverse plant community provides various habitats and resources for wildlife, enhancing the overall health of the ecosystem. For example, different herb species may attract specific pollinators, ensuring that these essential creatures thrive and continue their crucial work in the ecosystem (Katumo et al., 2022).

Native vs. Non-Native Species

When we explore sustainable herbal practices, choosing to focus on native herbs brings a multitude of advantages. These plants have evolved to thrive in their local habitats, which enhances their ability to withstand local pests, diseases, and varying weather patterns. As a result, they generally demand less upkeep, eliminating the need for frequent watering and pesticide treatments that non-native varieties often require. By cultivating native herbs, you can minimize your ecological footprint while fostering a more vibrant and balanced ecosystem.

Non-native species, on the other hand, often require more resources to thrive. They may need additional water, fertilizers, or pest control measures, which can strain local resources and harm the environment. Additionally, some non-native plants become invasive, spreading uncontrollably and outcompeting native species for resources. This can lead to reduced biodiversity and the disruption of local ecosystems.

Planting for Pollinators

Creating herb gardens that serve as habitats for pollinators is an effective way to enhance biodiversity. Pollinators, such as bees, butterflies, and even some bird species, play a vital role in the reproduction of many plants. By transferring pollen from one flower to another, they enable plants to produce fruits and seeds. Without pollinators, many plants would struggle to reproduce, leading to a decline in plant diversity and ecosystem health (Katumo et al., 2022).

To bolster pollinator populations, consider planting a diverse array of flowering herbs that thrive at different intervals throughout the year. This approach guarantees that pollinators benefit from a steady food supply during the growing season. Favorable options include lavender, thyme, echinacea, and rosemary, all of which are nectar-rich and draw numerous pollinator species. Moreover, eliminating pesticides and harmful chemicals from your garden helps safeguard these important creatures from toxic exposure.

Establishing a welcoming environment for pollinators also requires the inclusion of shelter and nesting options. Designating areas with bare earth, decaying wood, or small leaf piles can create ideal habitats for various species. Providing shallow dishes filled with pebbles offers essential water sources, aiding their survival during dry spells.

Guideline: When planting for pollinators, choose native herbs whenever possible, as they are better suited to local pollinator species and their needs.

Community Involvement in Preservation

Engaging in local initiatives is another powerful way to support biodiversity through herbal practices. Community involvement can take many forms, such as participating in workshops, joining seed exchanges, or taking part in conservation efforts. These activities not only promote biodiversity but also educate and inspire others to adopt sustainable practices as these sessions equip you with essential knowledge and hands-on skills, enabling them to foster beneficial transformations in their gardens and local communities.

Seed exchanges serve as another powerful tool for enhancing biodiversity. By distributing seeds from locally adapted and heirloom varieties, participants can play a vital role in safeguarding genetic diversity and bolstering the resilience of plant populations. Such exchanges cultivate community spirit and collaboration, motivating people to share resources and expertise for the greater good.

Conservation initiatives, including habitat restoration efforts, are also essential for preserving biodiversity where you can dedicate your time to rejuvenating native plant populations, eradicating invasive species, and crafting wildlife habitats. These initiatives not only contribute to the health of the ecosystem but also exemplify the significant influence of collective action.

Guideline: When engaging in community initiatives, seek out and support organizations and projects that prioritize native plant conservation and sustainable practices.

This chapter has highlighted the importance of ethical sourcing and environmental responsibility in the world of herbal remedies. By focusing on sustainable harvesting techniques, we ensure the resilience of plant populations and the long-term availability of natural resources. As we now move into the final chapter you will get an understanding of how these sustainable and ethical practices can be woven into your everyday routines. This integration not only enhances personal health and wellness but also reflects a broader commitment to sustainability and ethical living. By understanding the role of herbs in modern life, you can cultivate a holistic approach that respects both nature and human health, creating a harmonious balance between tradition and contemporary lifestyles—and that is what the coming chapter will be all about.

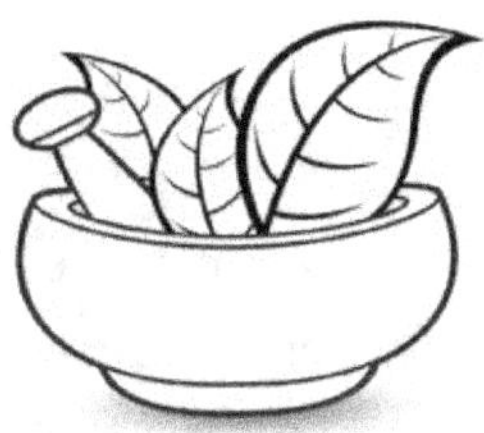

CHAPTER 9

Integrating Herbs Into Modern Life

Integrating herbs into modern living is not just a trend; it's an enriching journey that connects us with the wisdom of ancient practices. In this last chapter, we will explore how ancient herbal knowledge can enhance modern healthcare, thus creating a comprehensive view of health and wellness. For centuries, herbs have been essential to various cultures, prized for their healing qualities. Their revival in our fast-paced society highlights an increasing shift towards natural, holistic options that coexist with traditional medicines. Integrating herbs does not, however, mean abandoning modern healthcare practices. Instead, it can complement them effectively. The combination of herbs with conventional treatments can create a more rounded approach to health.

Blending Herbal Traditions With Modern Medicine

In our rapidly evolving world, combining the time-honored knowledge of herbal treatments with contemporary medical methods creates a comprehensive approach to wellness. This fusion can foster improved health and empower individuals to take charge of their wellness journeys. By exploring how herbal treatments can complement conventional medicine, engaging in meaningful conversations about herbal options with healthcare professionals, and acknowledging the research backing herbal benefits, people gain the insight needed to make well-informed health decisions.

When used carefully, herbal treatments can enhance traditional medical practices, providing extra support. To successfully incorporate herbal remedies into your healthcare routine, it is important to have open conversations with your healthcare providers, and engaging with healthcare providers about your natural remedies can be an approachable experience. Start by exploring the herbs you are interested in and gather solid information from trustworthy sources about their advantages and possible drawbacks. Articulate your goals and explain why you want to include these solutions in your health routine. Working together, where both you and your provider contribute to the decision-making process, fosters a supportive relationship and encourages a well-rounded, integrative perspective on health care.

Many people have found tremendous advantages in integrating herbs into their wellness practices. Consider Jane, a woman in her forties dealing with persistent migraines. While traditional treatments offered some help, the associated side effects were often overwhelming. After speaking with her doctor, she turned to feverfew, an herb celebrated for its effectiveness in alleviating migraines. She experienced a marked decrease in both the number and intensity of her migraines, which significantly enhanced her overall well-being. Another example is Tom, who battled anxiety for many years. Following a conversation with his healthcare provider, he began adding valerian root to his prescribed regimen. This combination allowed him to better navigate his anxiety, leading to fewer instances of crippling stress.

Herbal remedies are gaining recognition not just through personal stories but also solid scientific evidence. A study (Wilt et al., 1998) found that saw palmetto effectively alleviates symptoms of benign prostatic hyperplasia (BPH) in men, matching the results seen with standard medications. Moreover, research indicates that echinacea can enhance immune function and lessen the length and intensity of cold symptoms.

This highlights the need to incorporate scientifically backed herbal solutions into our modern health approaches, while still carefully evaluating their effectiveness (Hassen et al., 2022).

However, it is important to note that not all claims surrounding herbal remedies are supported by rigorous scientific evidence. The growing trend of self-medication with herbal supplements, often driven by misconceptions about their safety and efficacy, can pose significant health risks. Misbranded products, toxic ingredients, and lack of regulation contribute to these risks. Therefore, you must stay informed and cautious when selecting and using herbal supplements, ensuring that you rely on products backed by reliable research and manufactured by reputable companies.

Utilizing Herbs in Everyday Cooking

Incorporating herbs into your meals can be a delightful way to enhance both flavor and health. Herbs have the remarkable ability to elevate the taste of food, adding vibrancy without the need for added salt or fat. This not only makes your dishes more flavorful but also healthier.

Take basil, for instance. Fresh basil leaves can transform a simple tomato salad into a culinary delight, providing a burst of freshness that is hard to replicate with other seasonings. Similarly, rosemary can add depth to roasted vegetables, bringing out their natural sweetness and creating a robust, aromatic experience. The beauty of using herbs lies in their versatility; from parsley to thyme, each herb brings its unique profile to the table, ensuring that you're never short on options when it comes to enhancing the flavor of your meals.

Beyond their culinary appeal, herbs are packed with health benefits, as you are well aware by now. For example, oregano is known for its high levels of antioxidants, which can help reduce inflammation and support overall health (Opara & Chohan, 2014). In addition, herbs like turmeric have been praised for their anti-inflammatory properties, which can aid in managing chronic conditions such as arthritis (*5 Herbs and Spices*, 2023). These small but mighty plants pack a nutritional punch, making them an excellent addition to any diet.

Using herbs effectively in the kitchen doesn't require advanced culinary skills. One simple tip is to pair herbs with foods that complement their flavors. For instance, cilantro pairs beautifully with Mexican and Thai dishes, while dill is perfect for seafood and potatoes. Understanding these basic pairings can significantly enhance your cooking experience. By creating your herbal dishes, you not only tailor meals to your taste preferences but also make cooking a more enjoyable and empowering experience.

Creating an Herbal Home Apothecary

Creating your herbal home apothecary is both a fulfilling and practical journey, putting natural remedies at your fingertips for daily health and wellness. A thoughtfully designed apothecary fosters an active commitment to your well-being, merging time-honored herbal knowledge with the ease of contemporary life. This section will walk you through the crucial steps and considerations for establishing a customized herbal apothecary that meets your unique needs.

Essential Herbs for a Home Apothecary

Building a home apothecary begins with selecting essential herbs tailored to your needs. Think of your lifestyle, common health issues, and the types of ailments you might want to address. Here are some versatile herbs to consider:

1. **Chamomile**: Known for its calming properties, chamomile is excellent for reducing anxiety, soothing digestive issues, and promoting sleep.

2. **Ginger**: A powerhouse of anti-inflammatory and digestive benefits, ginger can alleviate nausea, improve digestion, and boost the immune system.

3. **Peppermint**: Great for headaches, digestive discomfort, and respiratory issues, peppermint is a must-have for its multifaceted uses.

4. **Echinacea**: Valued for its immune-boosting properties, echinacea can help ward off colds and infections.

5. **Lavender**: With its soothing scent and calming effects, lavender is wonderful for reducing stress, improving sleep, and treating minor burns and skin irritations.

6. **Turmeric**: Renowned for its anti-inflammatory and antioxidant properties, turmeric supports joint health and overall immunity.

7. **Calendula**: Used for its healing properties, calendula is beneficial for skin conditions, wounds, and inflammation.

These herbs serve as a foundation for a robust home apothecary, supporting diverse health needs and encouraging a holistic approach to wellness.

Storage and Organization Tips

Proper storage and organization are crucial for maintaining the potency and longevity of your herbs. Here are some practical tips:

1. **Containers**: Use airtight containers made from glass or metal to protect herbs from moisture and light. Mason jars, amber glass bottles, and stainless steel tins are excellent options.

2. **Labeling**: Always label each container with the name of the herb, date of purchase or harvest, and its uses. This practice ensures you can quickly identify each herb and monitor its freshness (Jessicka, n.d.).

3. **Storage Location**: Store herbs in a cool, dark, and dry place. Avoid placing them above stoves, dishwashers, or any area prone to temperature fluctuations and humidity.

4. **Organization**: Arrange herbs alphabetically by their botanical names or categorize them based on their uses (e.g., digestive, immune support). This systematic approach makes it easier to locate specific herbs when needed.

By following these storage and organization guidelines, you can create an efficient apothecary that not only looks appealing but also preserves the quality of your herbal collection (*Creating Your Home Herbal Apothecary*, n.d.; *Organizing Your Home Apothecary*, n.d.).

Understanding Basic Herbal Preparation Techniques

With your herbs organized and stored, the next step is learning how to prepare simple home remedies. Here are a few basic techniques:

1. **Brewing Teas**: Tea is one of the simplest ways to consume herbs. Steep 1–2 teaspoons of dried herbs in hot water for 10–15 minutes, strain, and enjoy. Common examples include chamomile tea for relaxation and peppermint tea for digestive aid.

2. **Making Tinctures**: Tinctures are concentrated herbal extracts made by soaking herbs in alcohol or glycerin. Fill a jar with chopped fresh herbs or half-filled with dried herbs, cover with alcohol (such as vodka), seal tightly, and store in a dark place for 4–6 weeks. Shake occasionally, then strain and bottle the liquid.

3. **Infusing Oils**: Herbal oils are useful for topical applications. Place dried herbs in a clean jar, cover with oil (such as olive or coconut), and let sit in a warm, sunny spot for 2–4 weeks. Strain and store the infused oil in a dark bottle.

4. **Making Salves**: Combine your infused oil with beeswax to create a healing salve. Melt beeswax, add the strained infused oil, stir well, and pour into containers to cool.

Learning these basic preparations enables you to harness the healing potential of herbs in convenient forms, making them easily accessible for daily use (*Organizing Your Home Apothecary*, n.d.).

Routine Maintenance of Your Apothecary

Maintaining and replenishing your herbal stocks is vital to ensure their effectiveness and freshness. Here are a few tips for routine maintenance:

1. **Regular Inventory Checks**: Periodically review your herbal inventory to check for expired or low-stock items. This habit helps you stay aware of which herbs need replenishing.

2. **Replenishing Stocks**: Purchase or harvest new supplies before running out. For frequently used herbs, keeping larger quantities on hand ensures continual availability.

3. **Monitoring Freshness**: Dried herbs generally last for 1-2 years, while tinctures and infused oils can last up to five years if stored properly. Pay attention to color, smell, and potency; discard any herbs that seem faded or lack aroma.

4. **Batch Preparation**: To save time, prepare larger batches of commonly used remedies like teas, tinctures, and salves. This strategy ensures you always have a supply ready for use.

By incorporating these maintenance practices, you can keep your apothecary well-stocked, ensuring that your remedies remain potent and effective.

Developing Personal Herbal Rituals

One of the most accessible ways to start incorporating herbal rituals into everyday life is through simple routines. For instance, establishing a daily tea habit can be a soothing practice, and preparing a cup of tea can itself become a meditative process, offering a moment to pause and breathe. Similarly, integrating herbs into bathing rituals can elevate one's self-care routine or align herbal practices with seasonal or spiritual occasions, for that fosters a deeper connection between nature and yourself. Each season brings a unique energy and set of challenges; aligning herbal rituals with these natural rhythms can enhance their effectiveness. For example, in spring, one might focus on detoxifying the body and boosting energy levels with herbs like nettle and dandelion. In winter, warming and immune-boosting herbs like ginger and elderberry can support the body during colder months. Similarly, marking spiritual events with specific herbs can deepen one's spiritual practice. Burning sage or palo santo, for instance, is often used for purification and cleansing during spiritual ceremonies.

You will want to make sure that you choose rituals that easily fit into your lifestyle, or else it will not become a sustainable and enjoyable practice. Your relationship with herbs will be unique, and finding what resonates with you can make the practice more meaningful. If you have a busy schedule, quick and easy-to-implement rituals like using a lavender pillow spray before bed or sipping on a relaxing tea blend during a work break can be highly effective. On the other hand, if you are one of those who thoroughly enjoy cooking, you might find joy in experimenting with fresh herbs in your meals.

Customization not only makes these rituals more practical but also strengthens your connection to the herbs. Engaging in a practice that feels authentic and enjoyable encourages consistency, which is essential for reaping the long-term benefits. Whether it's selecting specific herbs because of their symbolic meaning or adjusting the form of the ritual to match your preferences, personalization ensures that the practice remains relevant and supportive of individual needs.

The Future of Herbal Integration

The future of integrating herbs into our lifestyle is looking bright. Many people are turning to natural health solutions instead of relying solely on conventional medicine. As this trend continues, we can expect to see a significant increase in both herbal knowledge and its everyday use. This shift indicates that people are becoming more aware of the benefits of herbs and are open to incorporating them into their daily routines.

As herbal knowledge spreads, research into the benefits of herbs is likely to grow as well. Scientists and health experts are becoming increasingly interested in studying the healing properties of various herbs. This attention will potentially lead to new discoveries that could change our understanding of herbal medicine. By investing in research, we can uncover more powerful uses for herbs and expand their role in modern healthcare.

In today's health landscape, the connection between ancient herbal knowledge and modern medicine is becoming more pronounced. For centuries, different cultures have utilized herbs for their healing potential. A good example of this is Traditional Chinese Medicine, which emphasizes the use of herbs in treating various health issues. As more people learn about these ancient practices, many are beginning to recognize the wisdom that lies within them. By embracing this blend of old and new, individuals can gain a deeper understanding of their health. They can also act in a way that respects the traditions and practices that have contributed to our current knowledge.

Combining ancient herbal wisdom with modern practices enables people to take charge of their health in ways that may not have been possible before. For instance, a person can consult a healthcare professional while also learning about herbal remedies from books or reputable online sources. This dual approach allows people to make informed decisions about their health. A partnership between healthcare providers and herbal knowledge can empower individuals to manage their health actively.

This herbal revival is not happening in isolation. Social media plays a significant role in increasing awareness of herbal remedies. Many people share their experiences with herbs and the positive effects they have had. For example, blogs and social media posts often highlight simple recipes for making herbal teas or using fresh herbs in cooking. This grassroots movement helps normalize the use of herbs in daily life and encourages others to look into their benefits. As more people join this conversation, the collective knowledge about herbs will only continue to grow, leading to wider acceptance and understanding.

Moreover, educational opportunities surrounding herbs are expanding, allowing individuals to learn in-depth about their benefits. Many community centers, local health stores, and online platforms now offer workshops or classes on herbal medicine. Participants can learn how to identify herbs, understand their properties, and use them safely. For example, someone might join a class focused on cooking with herbs, where they would not only taste different flavors but also learn about the medicinal qualities of each herb. This hands-on experience enhances one's relationship with herbs, making it more personal and meaningful.

The future of herbal integration is not only about individual practices but also about community impact. As more people begin using herbs, we may see an increased demand for local herbalists and businesses that prioritize natural health. This demand can lead to the creation of more jobs and opportunities within local communities. People may find themselves drawn to herbalism as a career, which can also promote a deeper understanding of natural medicine in society. For instance, local herbal shops can serve as community hubs, where individuals gather to share knowledge and resources about herbs and their various uses.

As we move forward, we'll likely witness various innovations in how herbs are integrated into our lifestyles. With technology on our side, mobile apps are emerging to help individuals track their health while incorporating herbs. For example, an app might allow users to log their symptoms and suggest herbal remedies based on their entries. This type of synergy between technology and herbal medicine can enhance how we perceive health and wellness in our daily lives.

As we have now finished up this final chapter, exploring how to seamlessly integrate herbal remedies into modern lifestyles by blending traditional knowledge with contemporary practices, it is now time for you to try your wings and implement what you have learned throughout this book.

CONCLUSION

As we conclude our journey into the world of herbal remedies, it is worth reflecting on how far we have come. What started as a curious exploration has transformed into a deep and practical understanding of the benefits of herbal medicine for everyday health. From the initial chapters that laid the groundwork by providing historical context and basic concepts to the more advanced applications we covered towards the end, each step has broadened our knowledge and appreciation of herbal healing.

Our journey has not just been theoretical for we have dived headfirst into practical applications, exploring how to integrate these herbal remedies into daily routines safely and effectively. Each chapter provided actionable insights, whether it was crafting your herbal teas or creating salves and tinctures for specific ailments. These exercises were designed to bridge the gap between knowledge and practice, empowering you to take charge of your health naturally and confidently.

Throughout this exploration, we have consistently stressed the importance of safety and informed usage. While the allure of diving headlong into the world of herbal healing is undeniable, it is crucial to remember that education and caution are paramount. Not all herbs are suitable for everyone, and factors such as dosage, preparation methods, and individual health conditions must be carefully considered. Consulting healthcare professionals when uncertain and conducting thorough research cannot be overemphasized. Your journey into herbal remedies should be one marked by mindfulness and respect for the power these natural substances wield.

As we part ways, it is essential to keep the inspiration for continuous learning and experimentation alive. Consider this book as just the beginning of a lifelong relationship with herbal remedies. There is always more to discover, new plants to learn about, and fresh ways to incorporate them into your life. Enroll in a workshop, join a local plant identification group, or simply spend more time in nature observing and appreciating the flora around you. The journey is as much about enjoying the process as it is about achieving specific health outcomes.

The path to herbal wisdom is ongoing, inviting us to continue learning and experimenting. As you integrate these insights learned throughout this book into your life, remember the importance of approaching herbal remedies with both curiosity and caution. Engage with the community, share your experiences, and remain open to new discoveries. Documenting your journey can provide valuable insights and enhance your understanding. Now feel free to embrace this opportunity to enrich your life and the lives of those around you with the profound benefits that nature has to offer. Your herbal journey is just beginning, promising a future filled with health, discovery, and connection.

Thank you for reading! If you enjoyed this book, please take a moment to leave a quick star rating for this author, and don't forget to check out the full library of interesting topics available in this author's library of work.

GLOSSARY

Adaptogen: Herbs that help the body resist stressors and maintain balance by supporting the adrenal glands.

Aloe Vera: A succulent plant whose gel is used for its soothing and healing properties, particularly for skin ailments like burns.

Antibiotics: Medications that fight bacterial infections by killing bacteria or inhibiting their growth.

Antioxidant: Compounds that inhibit oxidation; a chemical reaction that can produce free radicals and damage cells.

Anxiety: A feeling of worry or unease that can be alleviated by certain calming herbs like lavender.

Aromatherapy: The use of aromatic plant extracts and essential oils for healing and cosmetic purposes.

Ashwagandha: An adaptogenic herb known for reducing stress and boosting energy levels.

Ayurveda: An ancient Indian system of medicine that uses diet, herbal treatment, and yogic breathing.

Bioavailability: The proportion of a nutrient or bioactive compound that is absorbed and utilized by the body.

Chamomile: A flowering herb often used in tea form for its calming and anti-inflammatory properties.

Echinacea: A group of flowering plants used to enhance the immune system and reduce symptoms of colds.

Essential Oil: A concentrated hydrophobic liquid containing volatile aroma compounds from plants.

Evening Primrose Oil: An oil extracted from the seeds of the evening primrose plant, rich in gamma-linolenic acid and used for skin health.

Goldenseal: A North American herb valued for its potential antimicrobial properties, often used in herbal remedies for infections and digestive issues.

Herbalism: The study or practice of using herbs to maintain health and treat illness.

Holistic: An approach to health that considers the whole person, including physical, mental, and social factors.

Infusion: A method of preparing herbs by soaking them in hot water to extract their active ingredients, similar to making tea.

Lavender: An herb known for its calming properties, often used in aromatherapy to reduce stress and improve sleep quality.

Lemon Balm: An herb used for its calming effects and ability to improve mood and cognitive function.

Menthol: A compound found in peppermint and other plants that provides a cooling sensation and can relieve nasal congestion.

Nettle: A nutrient-rich herb used for its anti-inflammatory properties and to support overall women's health.

Peppermint: A hybrid mint known for its digestive benefits and cooling, refreshing properties.

Phytoestrogens: Plant-derived compounds found in foods like red clover that can mimic estrogen in the body.

Placebo Effect: Improvement in a patient's condition due to the belief that they are receiving treatment.

Poultice: A soft, moist mass of material, typically of plant material or flour, applied to the body to relieve soreness and inflammation.

Red Clover: A plant used for its phytoestrogens, which are beneficial for women undergoing menopause.

Rhodiola: An adaptogenic herb known for enhancing mental performance and reducing fatigue.

Salve: A smooth substance that you rub on the skin to heal a wound or sore place.

Saw Palmetto: A plant whose berries are used to treat urinary symptoms associated with an enlarged prostate.

Sedative: A substance that induces sedation by reducing irritability or excitement.

St. John's Wort: An herb used to treat mild to moderate depression by affecting neurotransmitters in the brain.

Sustainable Harvesting: Collecting herbs in a way that maintains the health and balance of the ecosystem.

Synergy: The interaction of elements that when combined produce a total effect greater than the sum of the individual elements.

Tincture: An alcoholic extract of a plant or herb used for medicinal purposes.

Turmeric: A spice that contains curcumin, known for its anti-inflammatory and antioxidant properties.

Valerian Root: An herb used to promote relaxation and improve sleep quality.

Vitex (Chaste Tree Berry): An herb used to support hormonal balance and alleviate symptoms of PMS.

Willow Bark: Contains salicin, which is used for pain relief and has anti-inflammatory effects.

REFERENCES

Agrawal, S., & Goel, R. (2016). Curcumin and its protective and therapeutic uses. *National Journal of Physiology, Pharmacy and Pharmacology*, 6(1), 1. https://doi.org/10.5455/njppp.2016.6.3005201596

Asher, G. N., Corbett, A. H., & Hawke, R. L. (2017). Common Herbal Dietary Supplement–Drug Interactions. *American Family Physician*, 96(2), 101–107. https://www.aafp.org/pubs/afp/issues/2017/0715/p101.html

Ball, P. (2006). *The Devil's Doctor*. Farrar, Straus and Giroux.

Bhattacharya, M. (2024, June 21). *What Are the Health Benefits of Magnolia Bark*. WebMD. https://www.webmd.com/vitamins-and-supplements/what-are-health-benefits-magnolia-bark

Berry, J. (2012, November 8). *Herbal Healing Salve Recipe*. The Nerdy Farm Wife. https://thenerdyfarmwife.com/herbal-healing-salve-recipe/

Blumenthal, M., Goldberg, A., & Brinckmann, J. (2002). *Herbal medicine : expanded commission E monographs*. Integrativmedicine.

Breus, M. J. (2018, September 13). *Is Magnolia Bark the Missing Link for Your Sleep and Health?* Psychology Today. https://www.psychologytoday.com/us/blog/sleep-newzzz/201809/is-magnolia-bark-the-missing-link-your-sleep-and-health

Brien, S., Lewith, G. T., & McGregor, G. (2006). Devil's Claw (Harpagophytum procumbens) as a Treatment for Osteoarthritis: A Review of Efficacy and Safety. *The Journal of Alternative and Complementary Medicine, 12*(10), 981–993. https://doi.org/10.1089/acm.2006.12.981

Brown-Samuels, K., Hailemeskel, B., & Fullas, F. (2024). Acne treatment using tea tree oil, aloe vera, lavender, and calendula: The perception of pharmacy students. *International Journal of Frontiers in Biology and Pharmacy Research, 5*(1), 042–048. https://doi.org/10.53294/ijfbpr.2024.5.1.0030

Chadwick, P. (2021, March). *How to Grow, Harvest, and Preserve Culinary Herbs | Piedmont Master Gardeners.* Piedmontmastergardeners.org. https://piedmontmastergardeners.org/article/how-to-grow-harvest-and-preserve-culinary-herbs/

Chen, S.-L., Yu, H., Luo, H.-M., Wu, Q., Li, C.-F., & Steinmetz, A. (2016). Conservation and sustainable use of medicinal plants: problems, progress, and prospects. *Chinese Medicine, 11*(1). https://doi.org/10.1186/s13020-016-0108-7

Chevallier, A. (2016). *Encyclopedia of herbal medicine.* Dk Publishing.

Cervoni, B. (2024, April 18). *4 Benefits of Black Garlic.* Verywell Health. https://www.verywellhealth.com/black-garlic-8612816

Creating Your Home Herbal Apothecary. (n.d.). Mountain Rose Herbs. https://blog.mountainroseherbs.com/creating-your-home-herbal-apothecary

Curtis, L. (2024, March 6). *10 Healing Herbs with Medicine Benefits.* Verywell Health. https://www.verywellhealth.com/healing-herbs-5180997

Daily, J. W., Yang, M., & Park, S. (2016). Efficacy of Turmeric Extracts and Curcumin for Alleviating the Symptoms of Joint Arthritis: A Systematic Review and Meta-Analysis of Randomized Clinical

Trials. *Journal of Medicinal Food, 19*(8), 717–729. https://doi.org/10.1089/jmf.2016.3705

Dietary Supplements for Immune Function and Infectious Diseases. (2022). National Institutes of Health. https://ods.od.nih.gov/factsheets/ImmuneFunction-HealthProfessional/#h46

Dietary Supplements for Immune Function and Infectious Diseases. (2023). National Institutes of Health. https://ods.od.nih.gov/factsheets/ImmuneFunction-Consumer/#h47

Drug overdose. (2012). Better Health Channel. https://www.betterhealth.vic.gov.au/health/healthyliving/drug-overdose

Dynys, J. (2019, May 17). *Healing Salve | Herbal Salve Recipe.* The Everyday Farmhouse. https://theeverydayfarmhouse.com/homemade-salve-printable-labels/

Ekor, M. (2014). The growing use of herbal medicines: issues relating to adverse reactions and challenges in monitoring safety. *Frontiers in Pharmacology, 4*(177). https://doi.org/10.3389/fphar.2013.00177

11 Herbs That Can Improve Your Sleep. (2024, May 10). Bearaby. https://bearaby.com/blogs/the-lay-low/herbs-for-sleep

Ethical Sourcing: Gaia's Approach & Commitment. (2022, October 19). Gaia Herbs. https://www.gaiaherbs.com/blogs/seeds-of-knowledge/ethical-sourcing-what-it-means-for-gaia-herbs-gaia-s-approach-to-ethical-sourcing

Ewumi, O. (2022, October 6). *Herbal medicine: Types, uses, and safety.* Medical News Today. https://www.medicalnewstoday.com/articles/herbal-medicine

5 Herbs and Spices With Health Benefits to Try. (2023, August 28). Otterbein SeniorLife. https://otterbein.org/blog/5-herbs-and-spices-to-try-this-autum/

Galan, V. (2024, May 26). *Sustainable Wellness Starts Here: Ethic Herbs' Commitment to Sustainable Sourcing*. Ethic Herbs. https://ethicherbs.com/blogs/ethic-journal/from-farm-to-you-ethic-herbs-commitment-to-sustainable-sourcing

Garlic. (2020, December). National Center for Complementary and Integrative Health. https://www.nccih.nih.gov/health/garlic

Ghasemian, M., Owlia, S., & Owlia, M. B. (2016). Review of Anti-Inflammatory Herbal Medicines. *Advances in Pharmacological Sciences, 2016*, 1–11. https://doi.org/10.1155/2016/9130979

Gladstar, R. (2012). *Rosemary Gladstar's medicinal herbs : a beginner's guide*. Storey Publishing.

Green, J. (2002). *The herbal medicine-makers' handbook : a home manual*. Crossing Press.

Harder, C. F. (2019, December 17). *Our Favorite Herbal Blogs, Podcasts & YouTube Channels*. Chestnut School of Herbal Medicine. https://chestnutherbs.com/our-favorite-herbal-blogs-podcasts-and-youtube-channels/

Hassen, G., Belete, G., Carrera, K. G., Iriowen, R. O., Araya, H., Alemu, T., Solomon, N., Bam, D. S., Nicola, S. M., Araya, M. E., Debele, T., Zouetr, M., & Jain, N. (2022). Clinical Implications of Herbal Supplements in Conventional Medical Practice: A US Perspective. *Cureus, 14*(7). https://doi.org/10.7759/cureus.26893

The health benefits of 3 herbal teas. (2021, October 21). Harvard Health Publishing. https://www.health.harvard.edu/nutrition/the-health-benefits-of-3-herbal-teas

Heidi. (2024, June 20). *Glycerites: How to Use Vegetable Glycerine to Extract Herbal Constituents*. Mountain Rose Herbs. https://blog.mountainroseherbs.com/how-to-make-glycerin-extracts-glycerites

Herbal Academy. (2015). Herbal Academy. https://theherbalacademy.com/

HerbMentor: Your Home for Herbal Education. (n.d.). LearningHerbs. https://www.learningherbs.com/herbmentor

Hewlings, S., & Kalman, D. (2017). Curcumin: A Review of Its' Effects on Human Health. *Foods, 6*(10), 92. https://doi.org/10.3390/foods6100092

Hoffmann, D. (2003). *Medical herbalism - the science and practice of herbal medicine.* Healing Arts Press.

How Long Do Dried Herbs Last? Shelf Life and Storage Tips. (n.d.). Texas Real Food. https://discover.texasrealfood.com/food-shelf-life/dried-herbs

How to Make Infused Oil. (2010, November 18). Autodesk Instructables. https://www.instructables.com/How-to-make-Infused-Oil/

Huddy, J. (2024, February 23). *12 Best Teas For Gut Health & Digestion | Nourish.* Www.usenourish.com. https://www.usenourish.com/blog/best-tea-for-gut-health

Indigo Herbs. (2014). *Thyme Benefits & Information.* Indigo Herbs. https://www.indigo-herbs.co.uk/natural-health-guide/benefits/thyme

Karsch-Völk, M., Barrett, B., Kiefer, D., Bauer, R., Ardjomand-Woelkart, K., & Linde, K. (2014). Echinacea for preventing and treating the common cold. *Cochrane Database of Systematic Reviews, 2.* https://doi.org/10.1002/14651858.cd000530.pub3

Katumo, D. M., Liang, H., Ochola, A. C., Lv, M., Wang, Q.-F., & Yang, C.-F. (2022). Pollinator diversity benefits natural and agricultural ecosystems, environmental health, and human welfare. *Plant Diversity, 44*(5). https://doi.org/10.1016/j.pld.2022.01.005

Kenda, M., Glavač, N. K., Nagy, M., & Sollner Dolenc, M. (2021). Herbal Products Used in Menopause and for Gynecological

Disorders. *Molecules,* *26*(24), 7421. https://doi.org/10.3390/molecules26247421

Leas, A. (2024, August 1). *The Synergy of Functional Medicine and Traditional Medicine: A Holistic Approach to Health.* Yoo Direct Health. https://www.yoodirecthealth.com/blog/the-synergy-of-functional-medicine-and-traditional-medicine-a-holistic-approach-to-health/

Loscalzo, R. (2023, November 22). *Manage Stress, Anxiety, and more with Magnolia Bark.* ReInvent Healthcare. https://reinventhealthcare.com/functional-food-facts/manage-stress-anxiety-and-more-with-magnolia-bark/

Marquesen, S., & Kagan, C. (2021, August 25). *Growing, Harvesting, and Preserving Herbs.* Extension.psu.edu. https://extension.psu.edu/growing-harvesting-and-preserving-herbs

Mutterspaugh, M. (2024). *How To Harvest Medicinal Herbs For The Most Potent Remedies.* Theherbalistspath.com. https://www.theherbalistspath.com/blog/how-to-harvest-herbs-for-potent-medicine

Newman, B. (1985). Hildegard of Bingen: Visions and Validation. *Church History,* *54*(2), 163–175. https://doi.org/10.2307/3167233

Nutritional Approaches for Musculoskeletal Pain: What the Science Says. (2022, February). NCCIH. https://www.nccih.nih.gov/health/providers/digest/nutritional-approaches-for-musculoskeletal-pain-and-inflammation-science

Opara, E., & Chohan, M. (2014). Culinary Herbs and Spices: Their Bioactive Properties, the Contribution of Polyphenols and the Challenges in Deducing Their True Health Benefits. *International Journal of Molecular Sciences, 15*(10), 19183–19202. https://doi.org/10.3390/ijms151019183

Organizing Your Home Apothecary. (n.d.). Blog.mountainroseherbs.com. https://blog.mountainroseherbs.com/apothecary-storage

Petre, A. (2020, June 18). *Goldenseal: Benefits, Dosage, Side Effects, and More.* Healthline. https://www.healthline.com/health/goldenseal-cure-for-everything

Pietrangelo, A. (2024, January 16). *Which Natural Antibiotics Are the Most Effective?* Verywell Health. https://www.verywellhealth.com/natural-antibiotics-8414343

Rachel. (2016, July 13). *How to Harvest and Dry Herbs for Storage.* Grow a Good Life. https://growagoodlife.com/harvest-dry-herbs/

Reporting Serious Problems to FDA. (2020, September 9). U.S. Food & Drug Administration. https://www.fda.gov/safety/medwatch-fda-safety-information-and-adverse-event-reporting-program/reporting-serious-problems-fda

Ruggeri, C. (2018, July 22). *The Top 101 Herbs and Spices for Healing.* Dr. Axe. https://draxe.com/nutrition/top-herbs-spices-healing/

Schiller, R. (2024, July 15). *Can Tea Help With Allergies?* Verywell Health. https://www.verywellhealth.com/tea-for-allergies-5197793

Shenefelt, P. D. (2011). *Herbal Treatment for Dermatologic Disorders* (I. F. F. Benzie & S. Wachtel-Galor, Eds.). PubMed; CRC Press/Taylor & Francis. https://www.ncbi.nlm.nih.gov/books/NBK92761/

Snyder, C. (2020, April 7). *Magnolia Bark: Benefits, Usage, and Side Effects.* Healthline. https://www.healthline.com/nutrition/magnolia-bark

Sharifi-Rad, M., Varoni, E., Salehi, B., Sharifi-Rad, J., Matthews, K., Ayatollahi, S., Kobarfard, F., Ibrahim, S., Mnayer, D., Zakaria, Z., Sharifi-Rad, M., Yousaf, Z., Iriti, M., Basile, A., & Rigano, D. (2017). Plants of the Genus Zingiber as a Source of Bioactive

Phytochemicals: From Tradition to Pharmacy. *Molecules*, *22*(12), 2145. https://doi.org/10.3390/molecules22122145

Shishtar, E., Sievenpiper, J. L., Djedovic, V., Cozma, A. I., Ha, V., Jayalath, V. H., Jenkins, D. J. A., Meija, S. B., de Souza, R. J., Jovanovski, E., & Vuksan, V. (2014). The Effect of Ginseng (The Genus Panax) on Glycemic Control: A Systematic Review and Meta-Analysis of Randomized Controlled Clinical Trials. *PLoS ONE*, *9*(9), e107391. https://doi.org/10.1371/journal.pone.0107391

Streit, L. (2019, August 14). *The 9 Best Teas for Digestion*. Healthline. https://www.healthline.com/nutrition/tea-for-digestion

Thomas, C. (2020, April 19). *15 Medicinal Herbs to Grow & Their Common Uses*. Homesteading Family. https://homesteadingfamily.com/15-medicinal-herbs-to-grow/

Visser, M. (2015, April 1). *Using Herbs: Herbal Tinctures, Glycerites, And Vinegars*. Growing up Herbal. https://growingupherbal.com/using-herbs-herbal-tinctures-glycerites-and-vinegars/

Wachtel-Galor, S., & Benzie, I. F. F. (2011). *Herbal Medicine*. Nih.gov; CRC Press/Taylor & Francis. https://www.ncbi.nlm.nih.gov/books/NBK92773/

Wang, H., Chen, Y., Wang, L., Liu, Q., Yang, S., & Wang, C.-Q. (2023). Advancing herbal medicine: Enhancing product quality and safety through robust quality control practices. *Frontiers in Pharmacology*, *14*. https://doi.org/10.3389/fphar.2023.1265178

Weil, A. (2011, August 1). *Magnolia Bark for Anxiety, Depression?* DrWeil.com. https://www.drweil.com/health-wellness/body-mind-spirit/stress-anxiety/magnolia-bark-for-anxiety-depression/

What Are the Benefits of Herbal Medicine? (2022, March 28). The Yale Ledger. https://campuspress.yale.edu/ledger/what-are-the-benefits-of-herbal-medicine/

Wilt, T. J., Ishani, A., Stark, G., MacDonald, R., Lau, J., & Mulrow, C. (1998). Saw Palmetto Extracts for Treatment of Benign Prostatic Hyperplasia. *JAMA*, *280*(18), 1604. https://doi.org/10.1001/jama.280.18.1604

World Health Organization. (2023, August 10). *Traditional medicine has a long history of contributing to conventional medicine and continues to hold promise.* World Health Organization. https://www.who.int/news-room/feature-stories/detail/traditional-medicine-has-a-long-history-of-contributing-to-conventional-medicine-and-continues-to-hold-promise

Zhang, A. L., Xue, C. C., & Fong, H. H. S. (2011). *Integration of Herbal Medicine into Evidence-Based Clinical Practice.* Nih.gov; CRC Press/Taylor & Francis. https://www.ncbi.nlm.nih.gov/books/NBK92760/

Zick, S. M., Schwabl, H., Flower, A., Chakraborty, B., & Hirschkorn, K. (2009). Unique Aspects of Herbal Whole System Research. *EXPLORE*, *5*(2), 97–103. https://doi.org/10.1016/j.explore.2008.12.001